How Your Child Heals

How Your Child Heals

An Inside Look at Common Childhood Ailments

Christopher M. Johnson, MD

ROWMAN & LITTLEFIELD PUBLISHERS, INC.
Lanham • Boulder • New York • Toronto • Plymouth, UK

Published by Rowman & Littlefield Publishers, Inc.
A wholly owned subsidiary of The Rowman & Littlefield Publishing Group, Inc.
4501 Forbes Boulevard, Suite 200, Lanham, Maryland 20706
http://www.rowmanlittlefield.com

Estover Road, Plymouth PL6 7PY, United Kingdom

British Library Cataloguing in Publication Information Available

Library of Congress Cataloging-in-Publication Data

Johnson, Christopher M.
  How your child heals : an inside look at common childhood ailments /
Christopher M. Johnson.
     p. cm.
  Includes index.
  ISBN 978-1-4422-0203-0 (cloth : alk. paper) — ISBN 978-1-4422-0205-4
(electronic)
  1. Children—Health and hygiene—Popular works. 2. Healing—Popular works.
3. Pediatrics—Popular works. I. Title.
  RJ61.J65 2010
  618.92—dc22   2009050220

©™ The paper used in this publication meets the minimum requirements of
American National Standard for Information Sciences—Permanence of Paper
for Printed Library Materials, ANSI/NISO Z39.48-1992.

Printed in the United States of America

Contents

Acknowledgments

$\mathcal{I}$ thank my wife, Jennie, for her encouragement to write about the little people I care for every day, and my able agent, Anne Devlin, for her faith in my ability to write these books. I especially thank Dr. Kathy Rhodes, whose enthusiasm and skill inspired me, thirty-five years ago, to spend my career doing this.

Introduction

$\mathcal{I}$have watched children heal from illness and injury for more than thirty years. Throughout that time, I often found myself wondering just what, exactly, healing meant. We grown-ups stand over a sick child and watch the process, but really we are a far distance away from the actual drama, which is inside the child. There, events we dimly understand and barely control work themselves out. Ever since my first years in medicine, I have tried to imagine what the excitement and pageantry of those microscopic events must be like, because to understand them is to understand how healing happens. Throughout my years in the research laboratory, when I looked through the microscope I often conjured up scenes of the actors in the tiny drama unfolding below. I wished somehow to be there—if not as a participant, then at least as an observer. This book is my attempt to put you there, to share with you how those fascinating, complex events appear to me.

In the process, I skip lightly over a vast amount of medical research in immunology, pathology, and general cell biology. Other experts in these fields will likely find my brush too broad at times. But I think stepping back from the minutiae to see the forest for the trees is enormously useful. This book is a voyage of discovery into the astonishing microscopic world our children, and we adults, too, carry around all the time. It is a world full of wonderful, magical sights. I hope you enjoy reading about them as much as I have enjoyed studying them through the years.

1

Inflammation: A Visit to a Sore Finger

All children get sick now and then. Thankfully, nearly all of them get well, often as quickly as they became ill. Frequent, mild illnesses are part of growing up. So are the bangs and bumps children get, including the occasional broken bone. Such injuries virtually always mend with time. We take these things for granted, but we should not shrug them off without first acknowledging what they really represent—the wonderful process of healing at work. All those colds, earaches, sore throats, and stomachaches heal as part of a delicate chain of interlocking events. The same is true when the edges of broken bone knit together like new, or a cut rapidly becomes normal skin again. In spite of how complicated these processes are, they nearly always go off without a hitch. The fact is, children heal very well indeed. That is an astonishing thing, as this book will show you.

When you watch your child heal you easily see the outward events— the lessening of a cough, the disappearance of a fever, the drying up of a runny nose, the improvement of a painful sore on a leg. What you cannot see are the inward events, what is happening inside your child during the healing process. These inner events are the nuts and bolts of healing. If you understand them, you can appreciate just how and why, for example, that fever and runny nose went away. These are fascinating things to know. More importantly, they are useful things to know, because when your child is sick or injured, that knowledge lets you anticipate what tomorrow will bring. If you understand normal healing, you can understand what could be happening in those few situations when the natural process is blocked or interrupted and what can be done to improve matters. This book will equip you with that information.

Parents and physicians have watched children heal for millennia, keeping vigil by the bedside and worrying the process along. But it has only been in the last century that physicians began first to observe and then to understand the microscopic events taking place inside the child. The past two decades have increased our knowledge about healing exponentially, although we still have much to learn. The process has all the twists and turns of an epic production, although the major characters in the drama are on the order of a millionth of an inch in size. It has heroes, villains, stars, bit players, standard plotlines, and unexpected turns of events.

This book will make you a front-row spectator in the audience for a series of dramatic productions. To accomplish that, though, you will need to be small enough to fit inside the theater. You will undergo a virtual transformation that will shrink you to the same size as the actors. Properly miniaturized, you can then watch the drama unfold. Think of this book as a festival of entertaining and instructive plays, many of them interrelated. To take it all in, you will make a succession of expeditions, each of which reveals some aspect of how healing works.

Imagine this scenario. Using his father's tools, your energetic, twelve-year-old son has been busy constructing a fort in the backyard with scraps of lumber and leftover nails. After a few days of this, he complains to you that his left index finger is throbbing and sore. When you look at it closely, you see a quarter-inch size area on the side of his index finger, at the edge of his fingernail, is bright red. In the center of this red area, right up against the nail itself, there is a smaller grayish area. You notice the tip of the finger is more swollen than the corresponding area of his other finger.

Concerned, you call his doctor. These days being what they are, you do not get through to the doctor but instead speak with the nurse. She asks you if your son seems otherwise ill, if he is complaining of anything else, and you reply he is not. He does have various small nicks elsewhere on his arms caused by errant bounces from his efforts with a still unfamiliar handsaw, but these all look to be very superficial and fine under their bandages. Unlike the finger, they are not red and swollen. She asks you if he has a fever. You take his temperature and find it to be 98°—normal.

But even though he has no temperature, the red tip of his finger feels warm when you touch it.

The nurse tells you to soak your child's hand four or five times during the course of the evening and the next day in a basin of very warm, soapy water and call back if it does not get better or if he develops new symptoms, such as a fever. He will have to suspend the building project meanwhile.

After the third soaking session you notice when you dry his finger that the grayish area is gone and that the swelling and redness are better. There is a spot of cloudy liquid oozing out from the center of the red area. As the swelling decreased, and especially after the liquid came out, the throbbing pain got much better and soon disappeared. Over the next couple of days his finger continues to improve. For a day it still seeped a bit of fluid, but this was clear fluid, not cloudy like the first burst of drainage. After a few days, it looks exactly like his other one. He is ready to go back to hammering and sawing.

Sores like this are excellent examples of inflammation, which is the primary engine driving a wide variety of healing processes throughout the body. Since inflammation is so central to healing, a sore fingertip like your son's is an excellent destination for our very first voyage of discovery. The events you will see there are repeated in very similar form in many other places, following a wide assortment of illnesses and injuries.

Even though our detailed, microscopic understanding of inflammation is recent, physicians have known for more than two thousand years how closely connected inflammation is to healing. Ancient doctors had little idea what was going on inside the body, and the ideas they had were mostly wrong because they based their conclusions on fanciful interpretations of how the human body functioned. Yet in spite of those far-fetched notions, they did know some useful things. They learned these things by observing their patients carefully and noting the usual course of events.

Your son's finger exhibited all the cardinal signs and symptoms of inflammation, first described in Roman times. These symptoms are redness, swelling, heat, and pain. For centuries physicians watched for the proper progression and resolution of these symptoms as evidence that healing was progressing normally, even though they had no knowledge what the signs meant in regard to what was happening inside the body. They had some far-fetched ideas about it but only that. These days we can do much better. Every year brings new scientific insights into the fine details of in-flammation and how central it is to healing, a fact which should make us feel humble about ever knowing the whole story. Even so, we have a good grasp of what inflammation looks like at the tissue level and can confirm the ancient Romans were correct—inflammation truly is key to healing.

Now that you have had the full-sized, outside view of what happened to your son's finger, it is time for you to go inside to places where the ancient physicians could not go. It is time to take a seat in the audience of the microscopic drama. You are about to make the first of several trips you will make throughout this book in a tiny, imaginary, high-tech ves-sel. Think of it as a cross between a submarine and an all-terrain vehicle; it can swim in the bloodstream or leave the circulation system to crawl around between the cells of the body. It is well equipped with spotlights and spacious windows, allowing you to see what is happening all around you. The dramatic setting for your first foray is just before you called the doctor's office to ask what to do about it.

The blood vessels in the body form an immense, self-contained system that is divided into two halves. We need oxygen to live, and one half of the circulation, the arteries, carries oxygen-rich blood out to all the parts of the body, down to the tiniest places. The other half, the veins, brings oxygen-depleted and carbon dioxide–laden blood back to the lungs to get more oxygen, which we breathe in, and dump the carbon dioxide waste, which we breathe out. The two halves of the circulation join in a microscopic meshwork of vessels called the capillaries. This is where the true business of circulation happens, where oxygen and other important nutrients get delivered to the body's cells.

The capillary bed of your son's throbbing finger is the key place to visit as you investigate what is causing all the problems, but to get there you must first get inside his circulation. You need a location where the tiniest of blood vessels are accessible, close to the surface. The lining of the eye is such a place.

Imagine you begin by poising your craft at the base of one of his lower eyelashes. You look over the edge into the wet, shiny world below. Your son momentarily pulls down his lower lid, revealing the pink inner lining of his lower lid, called the conjunctiva. You seize your chance, zip over the edge, and find yourself motoring about in the clear liquid of his tears, nature's way of keeping our eyeballs moist. Here there are blood vessels close at hand, just below the surface. You slide your craft into the nearest one and then drift along with the stream, ever faster, as it takes you toward the heart.

You do not stay in his heart long, though, because nothing does. The blood rockets out of the heart like a fire hose, because the heart pumps an enormous amount of blood very quickly. A typical adult heart, for example, sends out about a gallon and a half of blood every minute, proportionally less in a child. The effect on your vessel is the equivalent of taking a trip over Niagara Falls. You get bounced around but soon find yourself in the aorta, the large vessel exiting from his heart.

The aorta is wide and fast, but it soon divides, then subdivides, into multiple rounds of ever smaller vessels. As this branching happens, the velocity of the stream in each of them slows down dramatically. Within seconds after leaving his heart you are scooting down one of these tributaries, headed for his painful index finger.

Things were moving so fast in the aorta and the first couple of branchings that you could not see any details in the surrounding walls of the blood vessels. Although you are going slower now, your pace is still a brisk one, and the flow still pulses along—now faster, now slower—in rhythm with your son's heartbeat. Soon the stream slows down enough for you to get some idea of just what kind of pipe you are traveling through. The first thing you see when you shine a light at the walls is a bumpy layer of cobblestone-like cells covering the surface. The junctions between these cells make a completely watertight barrier; no blood can leave this sealed pipe, and thus you cannot see what is going on in the tissues outside of it.

You soon find you are slowing down even further as you come closer to the sore on his finger, and you notice a dramatic change in the walls of the blood-filled passage you are passing through. For one thing, the wall of the tube is now translucent; you can shine your light right through and get a hazy view of what lies beyond. There are now some small gaps between the pavement of flat cells that makes up the walls, but the cells still mostly touch one another along their edges.

You have reached the capillaries. In real life there would be millions upon millions of options for you to have chosen on your trip from the aorta as the tubes branched into ever-smaller pathways, but for our purposes we will assume your miniature craft has the proper instruments to sense the correct path among the myriad of choices to lead you to the sore spot on your son's finger.

Before you reach the site of the action itself, though, you pause to look around at what is floating along with you in the bloodstream. It is a crowded thoroughfare because the diameter of the tube has become narrower with each branching of the way. When you were in the aorta and the larger arteries, things were simply shooting along too fast to see anything, but now the flow is more sluggish, and you can easily see your fellow travelers, the blood cells, out the window. Several of these cells are key to understanding how healing works, so this is a good time to look them over and learn a little about what they do.

You easily see there are two principal categories of cells. The vast majority, by a thousand-fold or more, are red disks with a dimple in the middle of each side. These are the red blood cells, and their only job is to carry oxygen. They accomplish this by being stuffed full, nearly to the exclusion of everything else, of a carrier substance called hemoglobin. When hemoglobin is loaded with oxygen it is bright red; when unloaded, it is darker in color. This is why oxygen-rich blood from the arteries is so red, whereas oxygen-depleted blood from the veins is a darker, reddish blue. The red blood cells go endlessly round and round the circulation, picking up fresh oxygen as they pass through the lungs and delivering it to the rest of the body. Healing body parts, such as injured fingers, require lots of oxygen.

Mixed in among the hordes of red blood cells, you see an occasional larger cell float by the window. Some of these are little spheres; others look more like jellyfish. Now that you are traveling slowly enough, you see that there is an especially large number of the jellyfish-type cells drifting languidly along the walls of the tube. Both the small spheres and the jellyfish are members of a family of cells called white blood cells. They are not really white, being more translucent in quality. They got their name mainly because they are not red and, when clumped together in a large mass, look whitish.

The jellyfish cells are called neutrophils. These creatures are moving along with you in particularly large numbers to your son's sore finger, because they are key actors in the cellular drama of inflammation. Although their walls are translucent, like a real ocean jellyfish, you see that they are filled with dark, granular pellets.

You and the blood cells have now entered the narrowest portion of the capillary meshwork. The passageway here is very tight, being the same diameter of the blood cells or even less, which must squeeze through in places by deforming and squishing their elastic sides. Now that the walls are pressing upon your craft, you can see that, as was the case further back up in the artery, these walls are also made up of cells stretched flat and stitched together along their edges like a quilt. Unlike in the arteries, however, here there are substantial gaps along the seams between the cells. These gaps are small enough that the cells cannot slip though, but some of the fluid part of the blood, the river you are moving in, does seep out.

Then you spy just ahead a strange thing: a neutrophil, one of the jelly-fish cells, has attached itself to the wall and is squeezing itself through one of the gaps. Neutrophils can slither and crawl along a surface, scrunching themselves between the tiniest of cracks between cells.

Finally you approach the scene. Your first sign of this is that the passageway walls have swollen back out, enlarged in size. This has created huge gaps in them. In fact, it is now difficult to tell if you are inside the capillary or outside it. The gaps are so big that quite a few red blood cells have floated out through the gaps into the surrounding tissue. There seems to be little distinction between the inside and the outside of the vessel. Since the walls are now as porous as cheesecloth, an even larger amount of the surrounding river of blood passes from the capillary.

What you are seeing from your microscopic window is the cellular basis of why an inflamed finger is red and swollen. Normal tissue does not have any red blood cells in it; they stay in the capillary network. The red cells function like long lines of boxcars laden with oxygen that pass through the capillary bed. As the train lumbers along it unloads its cargo of oxygen, which diffuses the short distance into the surrounding tissues to meet the energy needs of the cells there. Your son's finger is intensely red on the tip because so many red blood cells have leaked out, leaving their usual track.

The leaky capillaries also show you why his finger is swollen and painful—all that fluid leaving the blood vessels stretches the tissues tight as a drumhead. The pressure inside his fingertip becomes dramatically higher than normal, and the increased pressure pushes on the exquisitely sensitive nerve endings there. The result is pain.

But why did those capillary walls open up and allow all those gaps to form? What could possibly be the usefulness of having all the contents of the blood vessel leak out into the surrounding tissue? You drive on, hoping to find the answer.

There are still many red blood cells passing by your window, but by now there is a vast number of neutrophils, too. There are so many of these and they are all moving along with you toward the end of the finger that it is clear that these amoeba-like creatures are traveling along in response to a signal, a sort of bugle call, which is summoning them to the battleground that is the inflamed fingertip. The summons takes several forms: one comes in the form of substances given off by the germs invading your son's fingertip; another consists of substances that act as distress calls that are released by the cells living at the point of the enemy invasion; yet another comes from normal blood substances that are activated by all the cellular commotion.

The neutrophils are the foot soldiers in the inflammation wars. Most of the time they are called to fight outside invaders, like bacteria. They pick up the call for help, those released message substances, from the inflamed tissue and follow them exactly as a bloodhound follows a scent; like a bloodhound, the neutrophils can detect the concentration of these substances and keep going in the direction in which the concentration gets higher and higher, until at last they reach their target—the invading bacteria.

You are now moving toward the front lines of the battle, and as you get closer you pass many dead combatants. Bloated neutrophils are stuffed to overflowing with germs, bacteria, which look like tiny round clusters of grapes. The neutrophils have engulfed them, eaten them. When they do that they are called phagocytes, a word that even derives from the Greek word "to eat." There are other cells besides neutrophils that can be phagocytes, but neutrophils are the principal ones. Many of these cells are so full after their bacterial meal that they have broken apart and are merely drifting, dead after sacrificing themselves to destroy the invaders. The liquid around you is a murky soup made up of bits and pieces of cells and bacteria.

Those granular pellets you noticed earlier in the neutrophils are the bullets they use to kill the bacteria when they function as phagocytes. But as they fire off these bullets, the phagocytes themselves are injured beyond repair. Thus, a phagocyte is a sort of suicide cell that sacrifices itself for the good of our bodies. Fortunately, when needed, our bodies can pump out billions upon billions of these cellular soldiers in a very short time. This is why one of the most useful signs of an infection anywhere in our bodies is an increase in the number of neutrophils in our circulation. It is a test physicians use frequently.

Moving on, you explore the war zone a bit further. You suspect this is not a random fight, because there appears to be a method to the phagocytes' operations. Although as far as you can tell there is no overall, guiding hand—no single commanding general—this army clearly has a coordinated plan. The effect is very much like watching an anthill: at first glance, the ants seem to be scurrying around to no purpose, but if you observe them long enough, you can discern an organized pattern. By converging from all directions on the zone where the bacteria managed to get through your son's skin, the phagocyte soldiers surround and cordon off the danger area. A glance around the perimeter shows you how that happens. It is a marvel to see.

This battle, like any battle, has its front lines and its rear echelons. As the fight has been raging up front, you see that at the rear of the battle zone other participants have been busy. Behind the phagocytes there is a developing palisade—a stout wall—composed of tough, interlocking ropes. This material is called fibrin. It is also the stuff from which blood clots and scabs are made.

Fibrin is a solid material, but its building blocks are always circulating in the bloodstream, ready for use when needed. Several things can initiate the cascade of events that make the building blocks come together when needed to weave fibrin strands into a barrier. One of these is the debris of the fight, the bits of broken cells. Another is an impressive array of auxiliary cells—support troops—which answer the same call along with the phagocytes and join the scene of action. As the phagocyte·soldiers battle the invading bacteria, these supporting cells in the rear erect a defensive barrier to wall off and contain the battle.

How did those germs get through the barrier of your son's skin to cause infection? As you approach the epicenter of the action, you discover the answer. Sometimes germs can simply crawl through the skin via a small break, but other times they have an accessory to aid their attack. Up ahead you now can see that the bacteria gained entry to his finger through a break in his skin caused by a small wood splinter. The tip of the splinter stands in the center of the cellular fray, marking the spot where it began.

Like most battles, the outcome of this one can go either way. If the body's defenses win, the immediate result is what we call an abscess, a walled-off pocket containing dead phagocytes and dead bacteria. This is the whitish pus we have all seen beneath the skin of an infected area, such as a skin boil. Usually, there are also some living bacteria remaining in the pus, the relative amount of which depends upon how many were there at the beginning—generally, the phagocytes cannot kill them all. But any remaining living bacteria are now at least cordoned off, contained within the protective barrier walls of the abscess.

If the germ attackers win the initial battle, no abscess forms. Rather, the bacteria breach the body's initial defenses and spread through the body, sometimes by using the bloodstream, but other times just by marching through the tissues. When that happens, the child is generally quite obviously ill with fever and other symptoms, such as chills, muscle aches, and a general malaise. These symptoms come from all of those substances that got the inflammatory response going at the site of invasion—the signals calling the phagocytes and the auxiliary cells. Only now these substances are not just in one spot and exerting their effects there; they are circulating throughout the child's entire system. When that happens, it is usually a sign the child's body will need help dealing with the infection, such as antibiotic treatment.

The formation of an abscess is an immediate victory for the body, but it still represents a kind of standoff between the attacking bacteria and the body's defensive systems. The residual bacteria can still cause problems. For one thing, the toxins they release leak out into the regions surrounding the abscess and inflame those areas, too. Plus, the dead and dying phagocytes also give off substances that keep the fire of inflammation burning. For these reasons the area surrounding the abscess usually continues to be at least a little inflamed—red, swollen, and painful.

The bacteria remaining in an abscess can cause added problems, even though they failed in their first attempt to invade further. If they are still very numerous, they continue to reproduce, and they can do so very quickly—doubling their numbers every hour or less. Reinforced by all these new recruits, they can overwhelm the local defenses, break through the abscess walls, and spread throughout the body. One important thing that can aid bacterial growth is the presence of a bit of material foreign to the body, such as the splinter that is still in your son's finger. Phagocytes have a much more difficult time searching down and eradicating bacteria if there is something like that in the wound that gives the bacteria a place to hide.

You have now witnessed close up the complicated drama of what happens during what you may previously have thought was a simple matter—your child getting a small infection at the end of his finger. What you have seen are the early and middle stages of inflammation, the principal way our bodies fight off infections like the one on your son's finger. The same sequence of events happens on a larger scale when the initial injury and bacterial invasion is much larger. The larger the battlefield, the higher the stakes. For even the smallest abscess, a child's body usually benefits from a little help to handle the problem or at least to make it heal more quickly. Larger, more serious infections nearly always require help. So, having seen enough, you finally turn your craft around and leave the area. After all, you have to call the doctor's office to find out what to do about all of this.

What can we do for your son's finger? One very useful way we can help a small abscess heal is to open up the abscess cavity to the outside world. Often this happens spontaneously when the pressure inside the cavity created by the cellular warfare inside becomes too much for the walls of the abscess to hold. The weakest of these walls, usually the one facing outside the body, breaks and releases the contents of the abscess. This tips the balance strongly toward the body's defenses, because with a large amount of the remaining bacteria gone, the phagocytes are far more able to deal with the few that remain. Opening the abscess also relieves the pressure on the surrounding tissues, making the pain much better.

The doctor's office told you to soak your son's finger in very warm water several times each day. What this accomplished was to soften and break down the fibrin wall, weakening it sufficiently so that the abscess opened. (Larger abscesses may require that a physician lance them, a procedure called incision and drainage.) Depending upon the circumstances, such as how big the abscess is and its location, the phagocytes may require even more help in the form of antibiotic medicine, which kills bacteria.

A few days later your son's finger is completely healed. However, you do notice a few dry flakes of skin peeling off where the swelling was at its worst. This is because his skin was stretched by the swelling beneath it; when the swelling went down, it left behind some excess old skin that soon peeled off to reveal a layer of fresh skin underneath.

The process of inflammation made all this possible. You can tell from looking on the outside that everything is healed. But how did that mess you saw inside get cleaned up? Or did it? What does the next stage of the healing process look like inside, down at the microscopic level of the body's cells? This is as wonderful to watch as the events during the first hours of the infection. Besides the initial events you saw, inflammation is also a key mechanism in the cleanup of the microscopic battlefield. To understand that, you need to make another trip to see what the place looks like now, a few days later.

At first you see no differences as you travel down the maze of blood vessels toward your son's now-healed finger. When you get closer to his fingertip, however, you see that the small capillary vessels have sealed up again. The stretched out, cobblestone-shaped cells with all their edges stitched together, quilt-like, that comprise the walls are once again closely joined to each other. You no longer have difficulty telling the inside from the outside of the blood vessel because they are once again just tiny tubes for transporting blood.

Ultimately you get to the spot where the abscess was. Here things are definitely not the same as they were before. The first thing you notice as you approach is that the regular capillary roadmap is disrupted. Some capillaries end in blind alleyways, others split off at weird angles. What has happened here is that the original highway grid was disrupted by the inflammation. As the tissue healed, the capillary system had to remodel itself, laying down a few new roadways and sealing off others that were beyond repair. You have arrived in time to see the tail end of the project.

Once the little abscess was completely formed, its contents safely walled off from the surrounding tissue, the phagocytes inside it completed their soldierly job of eradicating the remaining bacteria. But when they were done, the place was a mess, littered and clogged with bits and pieces of cells and fibrin mesh. Soaking your son's finger in that warm water opened up the abscess and got rid of a good share of the debris, but there was still a lot left. Next comes the body's cellular cleanup crew to deal with the rubble.

Key members of the cleanup crew are cells called macrophages, cousins of the neutrophils. The very name of the macrophage suggests what they do: they are phagocytes, too, taking their name from that same Greek word meaning "to eat." They can eat bacteria, like the neutrophils-turned-phagocytes can, but generally they eat other things. They are like bulldozers that scoop up all the trash left over at a large construction site and haul it all away.

It takes you a while to find an open capillary that will get your vessel to the former abscess site, but after a few tries you find a brand new roadway. When you finally reach the site, you can still see a few macrophages crawling around, finishing their task. What brought them there? They were called by the same highly sophisticated intercellular communication network that first brought the neutrophils. Once the battle was over, the messages changed, summoning the cleanup crew.

When the macrophages are done with their job, it is time for rebuilding. Sometimes, especially if the spot of inflammation was small, as was the case with your son's finger, the cells in the region simply reproduce themselves and fill in the damaged area. The result is similar to replacing a demolished row house on a city street with a new one. After the rebuilders are done, there is little or no trace left behind that anything abnormal had happened there. Inflammation in which there were no foreign invaders—no microorganisms or splinters—often heals completely in this way, unless the inflammation was huge and extensive. Even then there may be no sign of what had occurred there.

Most of the time, though, there are at least a few spots where the battlefield cannot be replanted with cellular foliage such that no sign of the fight remains. This is particularly the case if the inflamed area was very large, such as from a bigger abscess. In those situations, the repair team must stitch together the boundaries of the battlefield and fill the hole left after the macrophages haul off the shards of cells, bacteria, and fibrin. The cells that accomplish this final step are called fibroblasts. As the last of the macrophages leave the scene, laden with their loads of refuse, you see the fibroblasts begin their work.

Fibroblasts are attracted to the old battlefield by the same amazing communication net that orchestrated everything else you have seen so far. The fibroblasts do not need to come from very far away. There are always a few of them around, scattered throughout all the body's tissues, lying dormant but ready to respond to a summons when needed. They do their main work once things have cooled down—the capillary vessels no longer swollen, the phagocytes gone, the bacteria dead.

At first there are only a few fibroblasts present, but very soon there are many more. This is because the cells that participated in or witnessed the battle release signals to the surrounding fibroblasts, instructing them to go into a reproductive frenzy. Soon there is a localized population explosion.

The fibroblasts fill in the holes. They also act like tiny ropes that pull together the edges of the old battlefield, causing it to contract. You can see the results of what fibroblasts do when you look at a healing cut in your skin—scars are made of fibroblasts doing their job. When they are finished, the tissue is as strong and functional as it was before, although it may never look quite the same. The larger the initial battlefield, the more this is the case.

Now it is time to leave. The macrophages and fibroblasts are nearly done with their work, and your son's finger, which already looks completely healed from the outside, is nearly healed on the inside, too. All this healing was orchestrated by the amazingly intricate process we call inflammation. But does inflammation always work this well? Are there times when it does not do the job? Worse, are there times when inflammation impedes rather than promotes healing? The answer is that sometimes inflammation is part of the problem rather than part of the solution.

As you saw firsthand, the hallmarks of inflammation are swelling, pain, warmth, and redness. In spite of the discomfort they cause, on balance these things are part of a healing process. There are occasions, however, when they occur spontaneously, out of the blue, for no good reason. Other times, inflammation—even though beginning in a well-behaved, appropriate manner—breaks loose like a wildfire. At such times, it can figuratively burn the whole place down, damaging normal tissue it should be protecting and helping to heal. Oftentimes these situations are caused by some external trigger, but sometimes the trigger is an internal one, intrinsic to the body, or is even completely unknown. You will read much more about situations like these in later chapters.

Inflammation is an intricate system. It is also a balanced one. As soon as it begins, the signals also begin for it to stop. The moment those first neutrophils make their way out of the newly leaking capillary vessels and start their work, other substances appear that serve to reverse the process. This is like a seesaw, a balance between forces that promote inflammation and those that reduce its effects. As the process works itself out, the things that block it progressively gain the upper hand over the things that stimulate it.

As you will see, there are some situations in which inflammation has an "on switch" but not much of an "off switch." Usually these situations eventually resolve on their own or burn themselves out, but sometimes we need to do something about it. We have several medications that dampen the inflammatory conflagration by closing the holes in the capillary vessels and preventing cells from releasing those substances that call other inflammatory cells to the scene. They calm the battle by interfering with the intercellular communication net.

When we consider intervening in the process by using medications that reduce inflammation, we are always aware of the fact that, on balance, inflammation is a good thing. It promotes healing, and, in fact, is a necessary part of healing. We rarely want to eliminate it completely.

・2・

Location, Location, Location:
An Ear Infection's Lesson

The well-known mantra for all real estate agents is location, location, location. That may be true for selling houses, but healing generally goes against this adage. Healing proceeds in a very similar fashion whether the problem is in your child's throat, her lungs, or her stomach. That is the great unifying principle of healing. Occasionally, however, this principle does not hold; there are notable times when location—the special aspects of a particular organ or place in the body—matters a great deal. This chapter will take you to such a special location to see an example of a situation like that.

It is midnight. Your two-year-old son has had a runny nose for a couple of days but has otherwise been fine; he has no fever, has been eating well, and has been his usual, playful self. That all changes when you hear him crying in his crib and get up to see what is wrong. When you pick him up you feel his flushed cheeks—he has a fever and he clearly hurts somewhere. Exactly where you cannot tell, although he keeps pulling at his ears. You give him some medicine for his pain and fever and both of you manage to get a little fitful sleep during the rest of the night.

First thing next morning you take him to the doctor. She looks him over, peeking into the back of his throat, listening to the breathing in his chest with a stethoscope, and pushing on his abdomen to see if it hurts there. She notices, as you did, that he has a cold with a runny nose, but that rarely causes such a fever and pain. She locates the problem when she shines a light into the dark hole of his ear canal, gently pulling on the outer part of the ear to improve her view. She tells you he has infection

19

in both of his ears in the tiny area behind his eardrums, called the middle ear. The fancy term for this common condition is otitis media, Latin for "inflammation of the middle ear." The doctor gives you a prescription for an antibiotic and also tells you to keep using the fever and pain medicines as needed. She says the antibiotic will take a day or two to work.

Over the next couple of days your son does get better. His fever is gone by the following morning, and soon afterward he is once again your happy, energetic son. A couple of weeks later, though, you notice he does not seem to be hearing things as well as before. For example, you have to speak louder to get his attention. Since he is just beginning to string words together into sentences, you worry his language development will suffer.

You take him back to the doctor. She looks in his ears again and does some tests that show he really is not hearing as well as he should be. The cause, she says, is a buildup of fluid in his middle ear. The first step in normal hearing is our eardrums vibrating back and forth in response to the sound waves bouncing off them. The doctor tells you that the fluid in his middle ear dampens this vibration, reducing his hearing. You are worried, but the doctor says not to be, because the problem usually clears up on its own. Thankfully it does, and a hearing recheck at the doctor's office several months later shows your boy's ears to be free of fluid and his hearing to be normal.

Ear infections are common. In fact, they are the most common child-hood illness resulting in a doctor visit, and three quarters of all children will have at least one ear infection by the age of three. Some children are troubled with repeated infections. For nearly all children, even those with more frequent infections, the problem disappears by the time the child reaches school age.

You and your son have experienced a common series of events, one familiar to many parents: your child got a common illness, after which his body healed. But, as with the case of the infected finger in the last chapter, what exactly does healing mean? You could easily see what was happening on the outside—his fever, pain, and subsequent hearing problem—but what was happening inside those ears, both when he first got sick and during the weeks that followed? To understand that, you will need to make a couple more journeys to see the microscopic drama unfold in front of you.

We begin our next expedition several days before he got sick. Imagine yourself miniaturized and seated back inside your tiny vessel, a combination submarine and all-terrain vehicle, with banks of windows on all sides to let you see all around. Your destination is his middle ear. Getting there, however, will require a roundabout trip. The most direct route would be to go straight in through his external ear canal, the place where the doctor shined her light to see his eardrums. Unfortunately, this will not work because the ear canal is a blind alley, with the path closed off at the end by the eardrum. You will need to get there another way; you will go through his nose.

Accordingly, you zip through his left nostril, taking the opportunity the instant he draws a breath. You have to move fast and keep your engines revved up high, like an airliner taking off, because the velocity of the air he breathes back out will be very strong in the narrow confines of his nasal passage—so strong it will blow your craft back out if you do not hurry. You also have to dodge to and fro to avoid becoming entangled in the forest of hairs that line the passageway. Even though the nasal hairs of young children are small and much less abundant than they are in adults, on scale with your present size, these hairs are tall as skyscrapers. Their job is to filter out and snag the largest particles of dust and grit we breathe in.

Skimming above the pale, pink walls, you see they are carpeted with what appears to be a fuzzy blanket layered with a soupy, shimmering coat of jelly-looking material. This is ordinary nasal mucus, and it has an important function. It is another defense we have against the debris in the air we breathe in. You can see it at work when you blow your nose after spending time in a dusty place. These are interesting observations, but you have no time to pause and investigate because any second your son will exhale and toss you back out into the room.

You also have to negotiate some other obstacles. The nasal cave you are in is becoming steadily smaller toward the back but not uniformly. It resembles a tall slit with walls made uneven by several large, bulbous protrusions from the side. As you whip by the first of these, you catch a quick glimpse of a small tunnel joining the main cavern. That tunnel leads off to one of your son's sinuses. The sinuses are air-filled cavities in the front of our skulls, and each one of them needs a connecting tunnel to let the air get in. Adults have several sets of sinuses, but in a child of your son's age, not all of them are developed yet. Having sinuses makes the anatomy of the skull more complicated, but if they were not there and everything in the region was solid bone, our skulls would be a lot heavier and much more of a burden to carry around. So they serve a useful purpose.

At the back of the nasal cavity you spy your entryway to his middle ear—the auditory, or Eustachian, tube. The opening is nestled right next to some swellings in the walls of the passage called the adenoids. Besides being a convenient way for you to get to the middle ear, the auditory tube is an important structure. To understand your son's ear infection you need to understand what it does. Now that you are here, it is well worth pausing to learn about it in some detail.

The auditory tube is a tunnel connecting the back of the nasal passages to the middle ear. Its job is to keep the air pressure between the middle ear and the outside world the same. There are tiny muscles surrounding the tube's entry point into the back of our nose that open and shut it when we swallow. For the brief moment it is open, air can go in and out, either filling the middle ear with air or releasing some of the air trapped inside it.

You can feel your auditory tube at work when you go up and down in an airplane. When you go up, the air pressure inside your middle ear is higher, in comparison to that in your nose, so some air leaks out of the tube to balance the two. When the airplane descends, air needs to get back up the tube, which is more difficult than letting air out. This is why many people are bothered more by landing than by takeoff. Marked differences in pressure between the middle ear and the outside world can hurt—the greater the difference, the more intense the pain. To help things along, you can make your ears pop—equalizing the pressure—by swallowing or yawning, since both of these maneuvers relax the tiny muscles pinching the tube shut.

You have been so busy navigating as quickly as possible to the auditory tube, the doorway to your son's ear, that you have not had time to give more than a quick glance at the walls, ceiling, and floor around you. Once you are well inside the opening of the auditory tube you are beyond the point where you might be tossed backward by your son exhaling or sneezing. It is a good place to take a break from the pell-mell rush of the first part of your trip, so you stop your craft for a moment in the apparent calm of the floor of this narrow tunnel to have a look around.

When you touch down, you plop into a gooey puddle of pale yellow mucus. It is not deep, but it soon coats the outside of your craft. When you shine a light out the windows, you discover your immediate impression was incorrect—it is not a calm place at all. Although you are out of the wind tunnel of the nasal passage, you are in a microscopic world teeming with all manner of bustling, tiny creatures—germs, bacteria.

The back of our throats and our noses comprise a veritable metropolis of germs of many different kinds. As long as they stay there, these inhabitants rarely cause us any trouble. They even do some good, by crowding out germs that can do us harm. In spite of this useful function, once in a while a new germ shows up and causes problems, such as the one that causes strep throat, but generally if the germs stay where they belong, our bodies coexist with them just fine. But how does that happen? How do our bodies keep the germs where they belong? On your present exploration, for example, what keeps them from crawling further up the auditory tube to the middle ear? After all, they are all around you now; it seems logical they would naturally head on up the passage, like pioneers looking for new land to conquer. To find some answers, you start your motor and drive up the auditory tube toward the middle ear.

The going is not easy. You quickly find that you are like a boat on the Mississippi, trying to push against the tide of springtime flooding, laboring upstream against a strong current. This current is generated by a forest of long, thin, hairlike strands sticking out from the walls of the tube into the stream, like a kelp forest on the sea floor. You would have seen these before, back in the nasal passages under the layer of mucus, had you the time to stop to look at the walls up close. Now, in the closer confines of the auditory tube, they are all around you.

The strands all beat in unison, like a coordinated group of spectators at a football game or a line of dancers at Radio City Music Hall. These amazing structures are called cilia, and they perform their back-and-forth dance to drive the thin mucous stream, like a conveyer belt, down the auditory tube and into the path of your vessel. Individually, each strand is a weak, trivial obstacle, but working together they generate enormous energy in the tiny world through which you are traveling.

As you make your laborious way along, you also have to dodge clumps of old, discarded cells and strands of broken cilia that are being pushed out, driven by the force of the mucous stream. The bacteria, you notice, rapidly becomes less numerous outside your window, and by the time you are halfway up the tube, you hardly see any more at all. As you get closer to the middle ear cavity, the mucus itself becomes thinner and cleaner, and the visibility is much better.

Finally, you pop through a tight opening and find yourself in the middle ear. You land your craft on the floor of this air-filled cave to have a good look around. In its tiny way, it is a majestic sight. Your searchlight reveals high above you, like stone arches in the Utah desert, a series of three delicately interconnected bones. The bones span the open space from one side of the cavern to the other. One wall of the cavern is formed by the translucent, pearl gray eardrum. When you shine your light on it you can see right through it, revealing some clumps of earwax in your son's ear canal beyond. You cringe a bit, wondering if you should have cleaned his ears out with a cotton swab. (The answer is no—never stick a swab deep into his ear canal. Gazing at the delicate structures around you, it is clear why: they are easily damaged.)

Shining your light back at the bony arches in the space above, you see the first of these bones presses up against the inner surface of his eardrum. The end of the third bone lies against the far wall on what looks like a tiny, oblong window. This structure has a matter-of-fact name: the oval window. There is another opening nearby, called the round window, because that is what it resembles. Both windows are covered by a thin membrane. Behind the windows lies the inner ear, but you cannot see it because it is recessed into the wall. The middle bone, directly above you, connects the other two bones with each other, linking eardrum to oval window.

What you are looking at is the astonishing mechanism by which sound waves in the air are transformed into a sound we can hear inside our brains. It works like this: when sound waves strike the eardrum, it vibrates. The vibrations cause the connected series of three bones to wiggle, passing the vibrations down the chain to the delicate membrane covering of the oval window. As this membrane vibrates, it causes the fluid within the inner ear to move. Sticking out into this liquid are the so-called hair cells, which get their name because they do look hairy; from the inner ear surface a matrix of delicate hairs sticks out into the liquid. When the liquid moves, the tiny hairs move back and forth. The hair cells connect directly to nerves that run into the brain, which finally translates these minute twitches and wiggles into what we perceive as sound. The little round window is necessary because, without its complementary movement in and out, the vibrations from the third bone pushing on the oval window would be unable to move the fluid in the inner ear. You cannot compress a liquid inside a rigid container—in this case, the rigid container is the skull bone encasing the inner ear.

The sensitivity of this chain of bones, membranes, and tiny hairs is another amazing aspect of hearing. It allows us to localize, quite precisely, from which direction a particular sound is coming. Our brains do this by comparing the intensity of the sound between our two ears: we can turn our head until the sounds are equal on both sides in order to locate the direction of a sound. This explains those instances when we find it difficult to localize a sound—in a cave, for example. Any situation in which sound waves are reflected off surrounding walls or structures can make them strike our eardrums in confusing patterns. We can twist our heads around to try to find the source, but if the sound waves come from several directions our brains will remain confused.

Hearing is indeed a fantastic mechanism. As your searchlights illuminate the overarching mini-cathedral of the middle ear, your son hears something, and you see the system function in all its glory—eardrum vibrating, connecting bones quivering, and the oval and round windows shimmering as they move. Inside the windows, you glimpse the hair cells waving. Suitably awed by the grandeur of what you have seen, you exit his middle ear and nose the same way you came in.

Hearing is an intricate system, one that can be disrupted in many ways. For children, ear infection is the most common middle ear problem, and your son got one of these. To understand what happened and why he got the infection, you need to repeat your journey, this time on the night of the fever. So you climb back in your vehicle for another expedition.

When you arrive again at the back of his nasal passage, near the gateway of the auditory tube, you find the place unrecognizable compared to your last visit. Before, the nasal mucus was so scant you hardly noticed it until you looked very closely. Now, mucus oozes off the walls in the form of yellow or greenish slime, carrying along with it clumps of discarded cells. The walls, ceiling, and floor of his nasal cavity are no longer a calm pink in color; they are an angry red, and they bulge out at you. In places, they even touch, closing off everything and blocking all airflow. When you make your way toward the opening of the auditory tube, you discover it is extremely difficult even to find it, obscured as it is by the swollen walls of the nasal passages and the thick gunk everywhere.

When at long last you do manage to make it into the passageway of the tube, you see that it, too, is swollen and filled with debris. In places it is completely blocked, forcing you to wedge your way through. The cilia, which before beat strongly and in unison, hang uselessly limp or wave back and forth in a feeble, uncoordinated way. The same germ-laden mucus you encountered in the back of his nose is here, too. There were germs in the first segment of the auditory tube on your last visit, when things were normal. But then the vigorous beating of the cilia steadily washed everything down, preventing the germs from extending their range more than just a little way past the opening. Now, stagnant puddles of germ-laden swamp stretch ominously out of sight toward his previously clean middle ear cavity.

You press on. When you finally reach his middle ear, after forcing your way through still more places where the path was completely blocked, you discover you do not recognize the place at all. Everything has changed.

On your last trip you found the middle ear cavity to be filled with air. You could fly about inside it or hover over the landscape below. Now flying is impossible—the air-filled cavern, with its intricate arch of connecting bones is no more. The middle ear is completely submerged, drowned in a murky sea. Now you need to activate your craft's submarine function, which it fortunately has. What happened here?

The explanation for this stunning transformation in the middle ear began with his cold, the viral upper respiratory tract infection he had a few days before his fever and earache. Common colds disrupt the natural defenses of the region. One key disruption is interference with the normal auditory tube drainage. For one thing, the tissues in the back of the nose swell, especially the adenoids, blocking the opening of the tube. For another, cold viruses stun the cilia, interfering with their normal, coordinated waving action. When the normal flow of mucus down the tube is interrupted, germs in the lower regions of the tube pounce, looking for an opportunity to do mischief.

Normally the bacteria living in the back of the nose cause no trouble—if they stay there. Germs, however, are creative and persistent creatures, and are forever attempting to break out of the confines of their normal habitat and find new body regions to conquer. There are several places in the body, including the back of the nose, where there exists a round-the-clock struggle between the germs and the body's defense system. The defenses must never let down their guard or malfunction. If they do, the germs quickly gain the upper hand, crawl up the auditory tube, and invade the ear in overwhelming numbers.

The first line of defense for the middle ear is the auditory tube's ability to beat back the germs continually trying to crawl up. Unfortunately for young children, several characteristics of their auditory tubes put them at a disadvantage in comparison with adults. Children's tubes are much shorter because their heads are smaller. This disadvantage is compounded by another problem. Adult auditory tubes have a kink in them and run downhill from the middle ear to the back of the nose. In contrast, children, especially small children, have a mostly straight tube, one that runs a more level course between the ear and the nose.

These mechanical peculiarities of their auditory tubes are the main reasons why ear infections are mostly a problem of childhood, although adults can get them, too. This is one important reason (and there are others) why doctors recommend that small children not be put to bed with a bottle: swallowing opens the auditory tube frequently and lying flat gives the bacteria a head start up their relatively short, level tubes.

With the auditory tube swollen and blocked off by his cold, your son's middle ear became a sealed-off space. Germs love a sealed-off space, especially one that was previously germ free. The bacteria, no longer held back by the normal mechanical defenses of the auditory tube, managed to swim up it and reach his middle ear. When they got there, they switched into overdrive, reproducing themselves and doubling their numbers as rapidly as every twenty minutes. Reproducing at that speed, a very small initial number of invading bacteria grow to many millions of germs within hours and to billions within a day. When that happens, the clean, air-filled cavity of the middle ear is very quickly flooded with a bacteria-laden soup.

You are floating in that murky soup, but you see you are not alone. Out the windows you see some old friends from chapter 1—the jellyfish-like phagocytes moving around everywhere. It is a familiar sight, looking much like what you saw in the infected finger. The phagocytes are stuffed to overflowing with bacteria, having engulfed and eaten them, which is their job.

Although you can see many of them swimming by, phagocytes do their best work when they are crawling on a surface, not swimming. Moving closer to the middle ear wall, you can see them hunt down the germs that are trying to break through the barrier wall and spread even further. Most of the phagocytes you see out in the soup are spent, merely drifting, stuffed full of bacteria. Others are clearly dead, even breaking apart, after having sacrificed themselves to destroy the invaders.

The inner walls of the cave of the middle ear have changed, too— dramatically changed. They are no longer a healthy pink but instead are red and inflamed. You aim your light at the far wall, the one formed by the eardrum. At first you cannot even see where it is because all the walls appear so uniformly red. Finally you locate the eardrum, but when you shine your light at it, you find you cannot see through it. On your last visit it was pearly gray, thin, and translucent; now it is thick and fire engine red. It even bulges away from you, pushed outward by the pressure of the accumulating bacteria and phagocyte-laden fluid in the closed space of the middle ear.

After what you learned in the last chapter, it occurs to you to wonder where the phagocytes come from and how they got there. After all, as you saw on your first visit, the middle ear is normally an open, air-filled space. It is easy to understand how phagocytes can get to an infected finger—they simply travel through the bloodstream, down the progressively smaller capillary blood vessels, all the while chemically sniffing out the increasing concentrations of the signals calling them there. How can that happen in the ear?

The answer is that the phagocytes get there in the same way they got to the finger—through the bloodstream. However, in this case they are working at a disadvantage. The inflammation in the middle ear sends out the call for help and the troops arrive, just as they did for the infected finger in the last chapter. But in the ear, they run up against a roadblock because they have no direct pipelines, no blood capillaries, that will get them in quickly and allow them to go to work.

Instead, they must squeeze between the lining cells of the middle ear wall, leap off the wall into the rapidly rising pool of fluid coming from the inflamed walls of the ear cavity, and start hunting for bacteria to kill. The fluid comes from the same process you read about in the last chapter—inflammation. Tissues in the throes of inflammation have a similar response wherever they are in the body: the cells in the area pull apart from each other, leaving gaps in the blood capillaries. Fluid from the bloodstream then seeps through the gaps along with the phagocytes.

Fortunately, the ear has other defenses besides the phagocytes, because relying on them alone for every ear infection would be potentially disastrous. The middle ear also can enlist in the fight something we call local immunity, meaning infection-fighting weapons located in the middle ear itself. One of these weapons is the combination of the coating of mucus and the cilia. Working together, both in the auditory tube and in the middle ear itself, these two help fight off infection by using what we might call mechanical means—ensnaring the germs and washing them away. The middle ear also has specialized cells living just beneath the layer of cilia. These cells release a specific kind of antibody that attacks bacteria (more about antibodies in a later chapter). The middle ear is not defenseless, even when bacteria make it all the way up the auditory tube to reach this normally germ-free sanctuary.

This is the point in the scenario at which your son woke up, his ear now painful and the flush of fever on his cheeks. His pain came from the pressure of the fluid buildup inside his middle ear. (You will read in a later chapter exactly how that pain happens.) Sometimes the pressure is so great it bursts the eardrum, filling the outside ear canal with infected fluid. This is not necessarily a bad thing. Although it often means there is infection now on both sides of the eardrum, relieving the pressure in this natural way greatly reduces the pain, and the drum heals in time. His fever resulted from some of the contents of that infected middle ear fluid being absorbed into his bloodstream and going to his body's thermostat. When that resets, the result is a fever, another fascinating phenomenon you will read about later.

Back in your son's middle ear, matters are at a tipping point. All of his ear's natural defenses are pushed to the limit. His body's goal is to wall off the infection and confine it to the middle ear, where it can burn itself out. Sometimes, however, the germs get the upper hand and reproduce themselves faster than the ear's defenses can deal with them. When that happens, especially if the cause is a bacterial germ rather than a virus, the infection can spread to other tissues, such as the bone that surrounds the middle ear or even to the brain. It can break into the bloodstream and spread throughout the body to other organs. Although these things are rare, they are always possibilities. Experts argue about whether or not the local defenses in your child's ear always need help to eradicate the infection and prevent such spread, but most suggest it is best that we give such aid in the form of an antibiotic.

Your child's doctor did indeed prescribe an antibiotic, and you filled the prescription as soon as you could because you naturally wanted to send help to the battleground of his middle ear as quickly as possible. But it is not as simple as that. Taking an oral antibiotic is a little like tossing a rock into a pond, and depending upon only the most distant ripples hitting the far shore to have an effect. It is a very long way from his stomach, where the antibiotic first goes, to his sore ear.

Before the medicine can help, it must travel to where the infection is. The only way for it to do that is through his bloodstream. Oral antibiotics are easier to give than are those that are injected with a needle, but we usually trade effectiveness for the convenience of swallowing them, because typically less than half the prescribed dose is actually absorbed from your child's stomach into his bloodstream.

Once in his bloodstream, the antibiotic circulates everywhere in his body, because the blood goes everywhere. This includes his middle ear, but it also includes places where no antibiotic is needed. Thus, a large portion of a swallowed antibiotic dose is essentially wasted. Enough seeps into your son's middle ear, though, to reach the place where the bacteria are busily reproducing themselves.

When the antibiotic does get there, the result is massive killing of the invaders, with the most actively reproducing germs being the first to go. The great majority of the germs are killed after the first few doses of antibiotic. This is because most of the antibiotics used to treat ear infections specifically target rapidly growing bacteria. However, there are a few of them, typically the ones growing more slowly, that can persist for a time. This is why it is important to give your son all of the prescribed doses of the antibiotic: we want to kill nearly all the germs, not just the majority of them. But even if the antibiotic does not get them all, and it usually does not, the combination of the phagocytes and the local immunity is enough to clear up the rest of the infection.

As I noted, there is some debate among the experts about whether antibiotics should be used right away for all cases of ear infection or if it is best to wait a day or so to see if the child's body can handle the infection without help from antibiotics. This is not an unreasonable approach since, as you read, a child's body is far from defenseless in this situation. Besides, ear infections have been a common childhood ailment since long before antibiotics existed, and children recovered from them. This is something for you to discuss with your doctor, although as of this writing, most doctors in this country advise prompt antibiotic therapy.

So, after a couple of doses of medicine, plus some medicine for the fever and the pain, your son felt much better within a day. By the time his antibiotic treatment was finished, he felt completely fine. But there was still the problem with his hearing a week or two later. What is going on in his ear now? Is it still infected? The best way to find out is to see for yourself, so you get back into your tiny explorer craft to make a return voyage, this time on the day you took him to the doctor for his hearing check. You again travel up from the back of his nose to his middle ear.

As you move into his nostril, quickly again to avoid being blown back out, you see that the redness and swelling of the walls of his nasal cavity are gone. Everything is back to its normal, pale pink color. The passageway leading back toward his auditory tube is wide open, although it still narrows as you proceed along. There is still a thin film of mucus coating everything, but thankfully the thick, yellowish-green gunk that got in your way on your last trip is gone. These things are all evidence that he has completely recovered from the effects of his cold.

When you approach the opening to his auditory tube, the first thing you notice is how easy it is to see compared to the last time you were there, when he was in the grip of an acute infection. That time it was buried in the swelling of the surrounding tissues, such as the adenoids, and did not open periodically like it should. Now it does, allowing you to drive easily through the orifice, after which you pause to look around. You quickly see things are better here, too. All the swelling, redness, and general oozing of fluid from the walls is gone. At first glance it almost resembles the tube you observed on your very first trip to the region, before he got sick at all.

Encouraged, you travel along, expecting to reach his middle ear without difficulty.

But you have no luck; after going only a short way you find your path blocked by yellowish, gluelike material that clings to your craft. This stuff is much stickier than the infected mucus you met last time, and is far more rubbery than the normal mucus you observed on your first trip, back when his ear was normal. With much effort, you slowly fight your way through the muck. It takes all the force of your engines, because the ropes of mucous strands are incredibly strong and difficult to slice through. A glance backward shows the gummy mess closing off the passageway right behind you. Previously none of your micro-journeys have been the least bit scary, but on this trip you wonder if you will be able to force your way back out—the goo is so strongly tenacious. Finally, after much effort, you reach your son's middle ear cavity.

The scene there is very, very different from your last visit. When you last saw it, the place was a battleground, a deep and murky lake filled with dead and dying germs and phagocytes. The place is calmer now and the walls are no longer bright red. But although the signs of acute inflammation are gone, it is not at all like the open, air-filled cavity you saw on your first visit, with its delicate chain of vibrating bones connecting the eardrum to the oval window of the inner ear.

The lake is partly drained and there are some bubbles of air above you, but the place is far from dry. Your craft is surrounded by the same material you fought your way through on your course up the auditory tube. It looks like the aftermath of an explosion in a taffy factory. The stuff clings to and drips from the bony spires overhead. The eardrum is no longer thick and red and it does not bulge as it did when the raging infection was present, but it is not normal, either. Now, it leans in at you, so much so that the middle ear cavity seems only half the size it was on your first visit to his normal ear.

On your first visit you had marveled at the delicate system of interconnected bones, moving in synchrony like the mechanism of a fine European clock tower. When you look at the caved-in eardrum now, however, you see it moving feebly in response to sound waves hitting it from the outside, and the vibration-transmitting bones connected to it hardly quiver—they are immobilized, glued down by all the guck. No wonder your boy cannot hear very well; the sound signals to his brain are severely dampened by the freeze-up of the mechanical conducting system.

All this does not look like normal healing to you. The injured finger in the last chapter healed up so well that, when you visited it later, you could hardly tell where the infection had been. Clearly, to be successful, healing in the ear needs to overcome obstacles the finger does not face. When you were last there, he had a firestorm raging, acute otitis media. The chaos you saw then was caused both by the effects of the invading germs and the efforts of two components of your son's body—his immune and inflammatory systems—as they struggled to beat back the infection. Your son's body, aided by the antibiotics he took, won the battle. But the battlefield is still a mess. You are glad his fever, pain, and swelling are gone, but clearly things are still far from right. What is this?

The proper name for what you are looking at now is serous otitis media. That is its fancy medical name. More apt, perhaps, is the descriptive term doctors often give it—glue ear. What happens now? How can this mess ever get cleaned up so that your son can hear normally again? The answer is that, nearly all the time, the mess does get cleaned up, although it can take a while. Over the years doctors have tried various medications to try to get it to heal faster, but there is no good evidence that any of these work very well. Mainly what is needed is time. The fluid will be slowly absorbed and the sticky goo cleaned up by the same cellular cleanup crew you saw at work in the finger. It just takes longer.

One key difference between a healing ear and the finger you observed is that there is virtually never any permanent damage to the cells living in the ear. There are no cellular gaps to fill or holes to stitch together. This means there is no need in this situation for fibroblasts, those healing but potentially scar-forming cells. Sometimes an eardrum that has ruptured several times from multiple infections can form a tiny scar as it heals, but ultimately this causes little problem if the middle ear can be cleared of fluid.

If we fast-forward several months later, you can visit your son's middle ear one last time. Now the pearl gray translucency of his eardrum is back the way it was; it dances as it vibrates in response to sound waves striking against it—vigorously for loud noises, barely perceptibly for soft ones, like a whisper. The connecting bones overhead once again wiggle like the mechanism of an old-style children's toy, sending signals on to the inner ear as they should. Your son has healed.

While we are on the subject of ears, we should consider another common form of treatment of ear problems in children, what physicians call tympanostomy or pressure-equalization (or PE) tubes, which parents usually refer to as ear tubes. What are they, and how might they work in treating ear problems in children? You now have a lot of firsthand information about the middle ear, knowledge that puts you in a good position to understand this issue. Bear in mind that the subject of ear tubes is sometimes controversial; they have a clear role in the management of some kinds of ear problems, but many doctors think they are used too much. I am not going to take a position on that controversy, because each child's situation is unique. But I will tell you the theories about how ear tubes work, allowing you to have an informed discussion with your child's doctor if that ever becomes necessary.

As you learned, the root cause for most ear infections is disruption of normal auditory tube function, and the most common cause of that is a viral respiratory infection, a cold, which clogs up the opening of the tube in the back of the nose. Children exposed to secondhand smoke also tend to get more ear infections, probably because the smoke causes chronic irritation and inflammation in the back of their nasal cavity. One way we know how important auditory tube function is for reducing ear infections is the observation that, although they are common in small children, adults rarely get them. We then couple this simple observation with the knowledge that, as we grow, our tubes get longer and run downhill from ear to nasal cavity, putting gravity on our side. The tubes also get a kink in them as we grow, making it that much harder for germs to crawl up them to the middle ear.

Colds are inevitable in small children—we get more of them during that stage in our lives than we do at any other time. One cold per month is common for many children. If the auditory tube is going to malfunction whenever a child gets a cold or if it chronically malfunctions for some other reason, is there some way we can help get its job done another way? If we can, perhaps we can prevent the resultant ear infections.

As you have read, the auditory tube has two jobs: the first is to let air go back and forth between the middle ear and the outside world, equalizing the pressure between the two; the second is to allow drainage down from the middle ear of the small amount of mucus and thin fluid that the walls of the middle ear normally produce.

The natural drainage of middle ear fluid is an especially important function for the auditory tube. If it does not drain normally, it can build up in the middle ear cavity. This can, by itself, mildly interfere with hearing. More importantly, persistent middle ear fluid is an excellent food for bacteria—they love it. Any stray bacteria that make it up the auditory tube to the middle ear are far more likely to win the battle with the ear's local immunity and reproduce themselves faster than the child's body can kill them, if they find there the friendly environment of a puddle of middle ear fluid.

Ear tubes are tiny bits of plastic that are placed across the eardrum, allowing air (and sometimes fluid) to go back and forth between the outside world and the middle ear. In effect, they are an auditory tube shortcut, a bypass. This allows two things to happen. To some extent, fluid that is in the ear can drain out. More importantly, the air can get in. The result is that fluid can much more easily flow down the auditory tube in the normal way. To demonstrate for yourself how this works, put your finger over the end of a straw in a glass of water as you withdraw the straw from the water—no water will flow out of the straw until you lift your finger off the end, allowing air in to replace the water leaving the straw. Ear tubes work the same way; they let air into the middle ear so fluid there can flow down the auditory tube.

Ear tubes do reduce the number of ear infections in children who get them a lot. By a lot, most physicians typically mean more than six ear infections per year. But it is not all gravy with ear tubes—they have risks. For one thing, at some point they fall out, and sometimes this is soon after they are placed. Another problem is that they not only let air in, but they can let germs in, too—in this case, whatever germs are living in the ear canal outside the eardrum. Finally, placement of ear tubes is a surgical procedure requiring a child to get an anesthetic, and that has its own risks, some of them serious. The bottom line is that the decision about ear tubes for your child is a complicated issue that needs to be individualized for the needs of each child and their family. There is no single, easy set of guidelines that applies to all children.

Healing proceeds in similar, even identical, ways across many different regions of a child's body. Those phagocytes you saw in the finger are the same ones you encountered in the middle ear. Sometimes, though, things are different. Sometimes the location of the problem really matters why things proceed as they do. Ear infections, with the peculiar anatomic characteristics of that region, are an outstanding example of why, on occasion, the real estate agents are right—it is all about location, location, location.

• 3 •

Sometimes the Body Does Silly Things: What Asthma Looks Like

Chapter 1, the story of what happens in a child's inflamed finger, gave you a view of healing as a well-coordinated, smooth process. First, the phagocytes and their helpers arrived quickly on the scene. Next came the battle between the finger's defenses and the attacking germs. After the battle was over, the cleanup crew, another sophisticated and well-organized team, did their job. Finally, the repair team made the tissue as good as new. All the players in these several acts knew their parts. The result was that everything returned to normal, and the reason that happened was that all of them worked together toward the common goal of healing. You probably finished the chapter thinking the body always does the right thing, following a grand plan, to restore health.

Reality is sometimes messier than that first scenario implied. There are times when the body does things for no good reason we can discern. At such times, we can hope nature is wiser than we are and knows what she is doing. It is entirely possible—even likely—that someday we will understand the body's reasons for doing what may appear to us to be silly things—or perhaps not. Until we know more about it, though, we are stuck with the fact that there are times when the body behaves in ways that are counterproductive to healing. In fact, there are times when the body's reactions to diseases and injuries are part of the problem rather than the solution. This chapter will make you a spectator to a microscopic drama that shows you an example of what I mean.

Imagine this scenario. Your son is twelve and has had asthma for several years. Everyone has heard the word asthma and knows it to refer to a breathing problem. What is important to understand is that asthma is not really a specific disease; instead, think of it as a way the lungs respond to a wide variety of things it does not like. These so-called asthma triggers include viral infections, dust, pollen, exercise, and many others. Although some of these things are frequent offenders, ones we commonly see across the spectrum of childhood asthma, every child with the disorder is different. What is a trigger for one child may not be for another.

Asthma is common among children, affecting around 10 percent of all of them to some degree, and it has become much more common over the past several decades. The reasons for its steady increase are unknown. Many experts suspect changing environmental factors, among other possibilities, but we really do not know for sure. Asthma is the most common chronic health problem in children, accounting for many missed school days and many trips to the doctor's office and the emergency room.

Your son's asthma is of the milder sort. It is not so bad that he needs to take medicine for it every day, but every couple of months or so he is troubled by its hallmark symptoms: difficulty breathing from wheezing, severe cough, or both. Today he spent the morning on a school field trip to the zoo and has been coughing ever since. Animals have never been a trigger for his asthma before, but things can change with this disorder.

Now it is evening and he is no better, maybe even a little worse. When he got home from school he was simply coughing; now, a few hours later, he is starting to have trouble breathing. He has had moderately severe asthma attacks before, but this one is the worst you have seen. You especially notice he has trouble breathing out, getting air out of his lungs. He is showing a common sign of this, one we use when we examine children with asthma—he cannot complete a sentence without pausing for breath after speaking only a few words.

Fortunately, you are always prepared for this situation. You keep at home medicine his doctor prescribed to inhale into his lungs to improve breathing. You give him a couple breathing treatments with this medication and he improves—he is able to move air out of his lungs more easily, and he says he feels better, less short of breath. His cough is better, too. You put him to bed after giving him one more breathing treatment to get him through the night.

In the middle of the night, however, he gets worse, and you can hear his loud wheezing coming from his room down the hall. You get up and give him another breathing treatment, but this time it does not seem to help much. If anything, he seems worse after the treatment. You are quite concerned; clearly this cannot wait until morning to call his regular doctor. So, in spite of the late hour, you take him to the hospital emergency department.

When you arrive at the hospital, the staff swings into action. They first give your son some oxygen to breathe through a mask because his lips look a little bit dusky and a probe they place on his finger indicates his blood oxygen is lower than it should be. They follow these with some additional breathing treatments like the ones you gave him and follow this with additional medications you do not have at home. They also give him anti-asthma medicine directly into his bloodstream through an intravenous line—a small plastic tube they place inside one of the veins in his hand.

All these things are standard procedure for any pediatric emergency department because asthma attacks are so common in children. The staff is also not surprised by the time of your arrival; for unknown reasons asthma in children often gets worse at night. Thankfully, within an hour or so your son begins to get better. This is also common; compared with adults, children are quick to get sick and quick to get better.

Now that he has turned the corner and is getting better, it is safe for you to leave him for a while and take a trip into his lungs to see what is going on there. You are amazed at how quickly and dramatically he got sick. The previous morning he had been completely fine; by the end of the day he was struggling to breathe. What is happening to him, and why did it come on so fast? As with your previous journeys, before you can truly appreciate what you are seeing in his wheezing lungs, you need to visit them before he got sick. So, as with the previous scenarios, you will make a trip down inside his lungs a few days before his class trip to the zoo.

You are once again buckled into your seat in your familiar combination hovercraft, all-terrain vehicle, and submarine. For this trip it is outfitted with a fancy new instrument, a device that lets you measure the direction and velocity of air currents outside the vehicle. Since the lungs are all about breathing and airflow, this instrument will be key to understanding how they work. The lungs are deep within the chest, and you have to travel some distance just to get to their entryway. The easiest course for you to chart is to follow the same route through his nose you used in the last chapter. So off you go again into his nostril.

You soon reach the familiar landmark of the opening of the auditory tube in the back of the nasal cavity. It looks fine, as do his adenoids protruding just a little out into the passageway ahead. Now you are entering new territory. The passageway makes a sharp turn, forcing you to dive straight down. The open cave of the nasal cavity has closed off here and you find your craft sandwiched between two sheets of pinkish muscle.

Pressing against your roof are the tissues of upper part of the throat, called the nasopharnyx. Pushing on your floor is what is called the soft palate. If you open your mouth widely and look in the mirror you can see your own soft palate—the soft flesh toward the back of the roof of your mouth, just before the back wall of your throat. The soft palate is easy to spot because an odd structure called the uvula, a kind of pendulum, hangs down from its middle.

Once you pass the uvula you find yourself in the back of your son's throat, heading straight down. You are getting closer to the entry to his lungs, but you still have some distance to travel. In particular, you need to navigate past the clever mechanism nature has devised to make air go to our lungs when we breathe and food go to our stomach when we swallow, without the two getting mixed up.

The windpipe, or trachea, is how air gets to our lungs. That is where you are bound. If you put your fingers on the front of your neck you can easily feel yours; it is a large tube, somewhat firm to the touch. The windpipe is easy to feel because it sits at the front of our necks. Food and drink reach our stomachs through a tube called the esophagus, which travels down our necks behind the windpipe. So air is in the front, food is in the back. To keep the pathways separate, we have at the base of our tongues a structure called the epiglottis.

The epiglottis covers the top of the windpipe. It functions much like a kitchen trash can that raises its lid when you step on a pedal. When we breathe, the lid opens, letting in air. When we swallow, the lid snaps shut, allowing food to pass over it and down the esophagus behind. Once in a while, especially when we are excited, we get confused and slip a little food or drink beneath the epiglottis; all of us have experienced the profound coughing fit when that happens. The epiglottis does a good job at keeping food out, but the lungs also use their very strong cough reflex as a backup system, just in case.

You are presently hovering at the base of your son's tongue, waiting for his epiglottis to pop open and let you in. When he takes a breath in and it does open you nip beneath its protective shroud. Fortunately for you, in your present state you are so tiny that you do not provoke a fit of coughing. If you had made him cough, the force would catapult you out of his airway and far out into the room. We generate enormous force with a cough.

Now you are at last approaching the entrance to his lungs, which looks like the entrance to yet another cave. (In fact, a useful way to think of several places in the body is that of a series of caves, places where things from the outside, like air and food, can enter and travel deep inside us.) This particular cave has an unusual door. It is not a round opening but rather a tall, vertical slit between two whitish pillars sticking out from the walls on either side. The pillars are the vocal cords. Their edges are not parallel, coming closer together at their tops like an arch.

If your son were talking at this moment, or actually making any vocal sound at all, the cords would be vibrating as he spoke. The way we make sounds is through those vibrations, which are produced as exhaled air rushes by them. This is why we cannot speak unless we are exhaling, usually slowly and steadily. This is also why it is hard to talk if we are having trouble breathing—the two go together. He is not talking now, which is probably a good thing, because at your present microscopic size, the volume of sound would be deafening here in front of his vocal cords. Although he is not talking, every so often the pillars move, snapping shut for an instant. This is a normal reflex we use to maintain internal air pressure in the lungs, which, in turn, keeps our lungs properly inflated.

You see that the force of the vocal cord gates slamming shut is substantial, and you do not want to be caught when they do, so you wait patiently for them to close, then open, after which you buzz quickly through before they can close again. Once you are through you find yourself in the long, straight tunnel of his windpipe. It is so straight your light can shine far down the path in front of you, and it is so long you cannot see what is down there.

Before you proceed further, you hover for a bit to cast your light about and investigate the world of the upper trachea. The floor is flat, but the walls and ceiling of the tunnel are supported and held open by a succession of arching bands of struts called the tracheal rings. The arches are complete semicircles, stretching from your left, curving overhead, and meeting the floor again on your right. They are made of cartilage, a stiff yet flexible material the body uses in many places where a semi-rigid support is needed. You can feel the cartilage rings in your own trachea if you press your fingers on the front of your neck. Other examples of cartilage support are your ear and the tip of your nose. In the trachea, these arches function like the timbers holding open a mine shaft; like mine shaft timbers, the tracheal rings keep the walls and ceiling from collapsing.

You find it difficult to hover too long in one spot because you feel your craft buffeted about in turbulent air. It feels as if you are piloting an airplane trying to land in a windstorm. But it is a strange windstorm—it abruptly comes and goes. One moment you feel a strong tailwind pushing you down the tunnel; the next moment you feel an equally strong headwind forcing you back. These to-and-fro gusts force you to shift power from front to back engines frequently in order to remain in the same spot.

What you are feeling is the force of your son's normal breathing in and out. All of us, even children, normally generate quite a strong flow of air. Doctors use measurement of this flow as a good way to tell how things are going with several different kinds of breathing problems, but measurement of airflow is particularly useful in caring for children with asthma. The precise numbers vary with the size of the child, but a normal twelve-year-old boy can manage a peak flow rate of nearly 10 cubic feet of air per minute when trying as hard as he can to blow out. That is a lot of air. A child can only maintain that flow rate for a few seconds because all the available air is soon gone from his lungs, but an air jet of that velocity is extremely strong. In your present state it would feel like a hurricane. Fortunately for you, your son is breathing quietly now.

Even though he is breathing effortlessly, the back and forth windstorm still makes you struggle to keep a straight course down his windpipe. One thing that helps you steady your craft is maneuvering it into a position right next to the walls, where the violent changes in airflow direction are much less pronounced. This also lets you get a closer look at those walls.

You see the walls to be pink, moist, and covered with a minutely fuzzy surface. You have seen this sort of thing before. When you peer more closely at this fuzz, you see it is comprised of the same sort of cells you found in the auditory tube of your other son's ears. You see the same tiny, hairlike cilia, all waving in unison like fans at a football game. As they did in the auditory tube, their coordinated efforts move along a thin coating of clear mucus.

In the auditory tube, the cilia-driven conveyer belt mostly carries back germs that are forever trying to crawl up to the middle ear. The same thing happens in the windpipe—bacteria in the mouth are constantly trying to get down into the lungs. The tracheal system, however, has a bigger, more formidable job than that of the auditory tube. The trachea must contend with much more than germs trying to sneak in the front door to the lungs; the trachea also must deal with all the dust, dirt, pollen, and everything else floating in the air we breathe.

You have already passed the lung's first line of defense—the nose. When sitting quietly we mostly breathe through our noses rather than our mouths, and many particles get filtered out there. For those particles that make it past the nose, the largest ones we inhale do not make it very far into the lungs because they are often big enough to trigger a cough reflex.

A good example of this is what happens when, out on an evening walk, you inhale a small bug: you quickly and violently cough it back out. In contrast, smaller particles like tiny bits of soot and grains of pollen (and your exploration vessel) do not provoke a cough, so they can travel deeply into the lungs with each breath. All of this debris needs to go somewhere; it must either be carried back out of the lungs by the mucous-cilia conveyer belt, or else be absorbed into the lung tissue.

The mucous and cilia scrubbing system is very efficient at keeping the lungs clean. Most do not realize it, but when you clear your throat with a small cough you are actually implementing the last phase of the process: the cilia have delivered a load of debris-laden mucus to the portal of the lung, dumping it out the door. You then cough it into your mouth and swallow it. Doctors occasionally take advantage of this reflex. We sometimes can find what is going on deep in the lungs by looking at what has made it into the stomach. So, although you can hover above the mucous blanket moving methodically along below, you take care not to get trapped in it, lest you be pushed back out of the lungs and swallowed with all the other trash.

Depending upon where your son has been lately, there can be quite a lot of debris for the lungs to unload. On your journey today, you recall that two days earlier he spent the morning playing behind the house with a shovel, digging a hole to China. He did not make it any further than three feet down, but you can see the results of the shovelfuls of dirt tossed into the air. There are globs of mucus all around you, like wet spackle on a wall, which are studded with grains of dirt. Between the globs the surface is smooth as it undulates back and forth between the overarching rings of cartilage.

As you travel down the long passage, you notice it is progressively getting smaller, until finally you reach a fork in the road. One tunnel leads off to the left at about a 45-degree angle; the one to the right is more straight ahead. You are presently at the spot where airflow divides equally between the paths to your son's left and right lungs. You pause and shine your light down each one—they look the same. You pick the branch to the left lung.

Once into the new tunnel, called the left bronchus, you soon feel the walls and ceiling moving closer to you—it is barely half the diameter of the lower end of the windpipe you just left. There are still those circular struts holding the passage open, but they, too, are narrower and more delicate. At least the fierce air turbulence you felt in the windpipe is a little better, but you still feel a swaying, back-and-forth movement as your son breathes in and out. The whole place, in fact, rocks and shakes gently with each breath; the walls, ceiling, and floor bow in and out with the natural rhythm of his breathing.

Your lights immediately pick out another fork in the road dead ahead, again with two possible routes. When you stop to consider which way to go, you look up at the ceiling of the bronchus and notice it is pulsating in and out in one spot. When you shine a light on the spot you see a shadow just outside the passageway. It is a large pipe that appears to be lying across the tunnel, pushing on it slightly from the outside. This pipe is a branch of the pulmonary artery, the huge blood vessel that leads from your son's heart to his lungs, bringing blood to the lungs to pick up essential oxygen.

As you pass down ever-smaller branches of the tunnel maze, you sense you are right next to his heart. It makes everything around you bounce along with his heartbeats, and you can easily hear the thump of his heart kicking against its surrounding tissues and the nearby whoosh of the blood passing through his heart's chambers.

You are now deeper inside his lung. The tiny passageway does not have those buttressing cartilage beams to support the walls. For a while after you left the midsized air tunnels, there was a cobblestone pattern of pieces of firm, supporting cartilage set in the walls like flagstones, but now those are gone, too. You are now in a bronchiole, the tiniest part of the air tunnel network. Here everything is more lax. The walls lean in at you dramatically with each of your son's breaths. Now the turbulence is gone. You feel placid air flowing gently in and out—all is calm.

You feel as if your passageway might close off completely, and although it comes close, it never closes. You have just made a very important observation. Since all these very small airways are floppy, not held open by any cartilage scaffolding to support the walls, it is vital that they not close off, because then no air could get in or out. What holds them open is the natural stretchiness, the intrinsic elasticity, of the lung tissue. Each little cluster of alveolar sacs of the lung has its own set of tubes feeding air to it. If one group of clusters becomes filled with too much air, the swollen region can press down on the small air tubes passing nearby on their way to bring air to other clusters, pinching them off. There are times when this happens, and it is always a problem when it does.

Down here the walls of the breathing tube network have changed their character in other ways besides losing their built-in struts. Now when you shine your light at the walls, you see they are thinned to near transparency. Through them you can easily see a meshwork of muscle cords surrounding the passageway outside, ropy bands encircling it at close intervals. You go on a little further, encountering airflow that is only a faint breeze blowing alternately forward and backward. Every now and then along the passage, there are little alcoves budding out from the wall like bay windows. The walls of these are transparent. You have reached a terminal bronchiole, the point where the simple air-conducting network of the lungs, the mass of ever-smaller tubes, reaches the true business part of the lung. That business is the exchange of gases.

We are, in a very real sense, internal combustion engines, like our cars. We use oxygen to burn fuel and produce energy. Also like our cars, the chief result of this combustion process is water and carbon dioxide. The lungs are both where our bodies absorb the needed oxygen for combustion and dump the carbon dioxide waste from the spent fuel. (We deal with the water that gets produced as a by-product in other ways.) Our lungs are both the air intake and the exhaust pipe for our human engines. Unlike cars, though, our fuel is not gasoline—it is the food we eat, which we "burn" through chemical reactions.

Those little alcoves, the bay windows you see in the walls of the terminal bronchiole, are the first sign you are reaching the place where gas exchange happens, where our bodies swap carbon dioxide for fresh oxygen. You travel just a bit further down the last of these passages and suddenly find yourself in a large space again. After the tight quarters you have just left, this is a relief, but you soon see that the room you are in goes nowhere—it is a dead end. You have reached what are called the alveolar sacs and can go no further.

You park your craft and shine your light all around. The place feels positively huge after the confining, tight space of the terminal bronchiole. Scanning your light on the walls, the ceiling, and the floor shows that you are in a kind of suite of round-walled rooms, but the rooms lack most of their interior walls. Instead, the chambers are all connected by wide openings. Here you feel only the gentlest of air currents.

The walls, floor, and ceiling of this cluster of rooms are spectacular to look at. They resemble an ornamental fountain, the kind in which a thin sheet of water slides down a smooth rock surface. But the liquid sheet is not water—it is blood. The walls are blood red because they are completely transparent. The only way you know the walls are even there is the fact that the blood gliding past around you, above you, and beneath you must be held back by something or it would flood down on top of you. Here and there you see areas of more solid tissue through the walls, places where your suite of rooms and the adjoining ones are tethered together, but your overall impression is one of a spectacular, all-surrounding, red river.

Small as you are, you still cannot see things at the tiniest level, that of the individual gas molecules, so you cannot see precisely what is happening all around you and in the millions upon millions of other chambers in the lung just like the one you are in. You arrived in the alveolar sac on a stream of fresh, oxygen-rich air. When you turn to leave your son's lungs, you will voyage back on a current of air laden with carbon dioxide that has changed places with the oxygen in the blood that is streaming in the walls all around you. The reason the walls of the chambers are so thin is to allow free passage of these gases to and from the blood—out with the bad air, in with the good. It is a marvelous system.

Having now reached the end of your first exploration of the lungs, you reluctantly turn your craft around to leave this spectacle. You motor out through progressively larger air tubes until mid-trachea when your son shoots you out his mouth with a sudden cough.

Now that you have seen the respiratory system close up, you are ready to learn what happened when things went wrong and your son had his asthma attack. The best time to begin your return trip is the moment when your son arrived at the emergency department. So let us leave him for a figurative moment in the excellent care of the emergency department staff and go take a look for ourselves at the problem in his lungs now.

When you approach his nostril you immediately see something different than last time. Before, his nose did not move as he drew air in; now, however, the sides of his nose flare outward with each breath. This is characteristic of children with all sorts of breathing troubles, including asthma. It indicates that they are feeling short of breath. Just before you go inside, you glance down at his neck where it joins the top of his chest. There, too, different things are happening. Unlike before, you see the base of his neck moving inward with each of his breaths. It looks backward to you, and you are right—it is a sort of backward breathing. Such retractions, as they are called, happen when a child is working hard to get air in and out of his lungs.

Once inside his nasal cavity again you notice something else. Things there are quiet—too quiet—because there is much less turbulent airflow. Once you get under the epiglottis and enter the trachea you find there, too, things have changed. On your previous trip, as soon as you passed between his vocal cords, you were immediately tossed and tumbled about in rapidly rushing air. It was like being in a wind tunnel, but one that fiercely reversed direction with every breath. You had to skim along close to the wall to avoid the worst of the storm. The turbulence did not relent much until you reached the second or third branching of his air tubes.

Now things are strangely different. You still feel your vessel pulled deeper into his lungs when he breathes in but not as forcefully as before. What is really different is that the onrushing headwind that once blew against you when he breathed out, expelling air from his lungs, is gone. On your last trip you met a wind that ramped up instantaneously in force from nothing to gale force with each breath; now you find yourself piloting your way against a steady and quite gentle breeze blowing up from his lungs.

There is something else you notice. Before, there was a pause between his breathing out and drawing his next breath in; it was a moment of calm when all air movement stopped entirely between breaths. That has changed. Now the steady, exhaling breeze blows unchanging against your craft. It is a feeble stream compared with what you encountered on your last expedition, and it never ceases until you abruptly feel a burst of air coming from behind you, when he finally must take another breath in.

What you are experiencing is one of the key derangements during an asthma attack—obstruction of air getting out of the lungs. Normally air leaves our lungs of its own accord, passively. When we are resting comfortably, it takes almost no effort to exhale. The intrinsic, natural elasticity of our chest simply pushes the air back out after we are finished drawing it in, similar to what happens if you open the spout of an inflated balloon. That is when we are at rest. If we wish, we can use our chest muscles to get the air out faster by squeezing them down on our ribs, such as when we are exerting ourselves. But most of the time, breathing in is active, breathing out is passive.

That changes in an asthma attack. Before you miniaturized yourself for the trip, you noticed your son was doing everything he could to get air out of his lungs, squeezing his chest muscles to force it out, as if he were squeezing on a set of bagpipes. He even sounded a bit like bagpipes, because the sound of the steady, slow-flowing air through obstructed air passages makes a characteristic sound, called a wheeze. It is a hallmark of asthma. A doctor or nurse can easily hear a wheeze through a stethoscope. In a moderate or severe asthma attack, you do not need a stethoscope because often the wheezing is audible across the room.

What is causing this obstruction of air coming out of his lungs? His upper trachea looks pretty normal, although you do detect a hint of redness in the walls. Now that you know the way inside and what normal lungs look like, you need to press on to discover the cause of the blockage. Once you find just what it is and understand why that is happening, you can understand how and why we go about relieving the symptoms of an asthma attack.

At first you do not see much that is helpful. His windpipe down to the first branching, and even beyond that point, is wide open. No blockage so far. You do notice some evidence that things are not normal. The velvety walls of the windpipe become progressively more reddened. On your last trip you had seen occasional blobs of thick mucus on the walls or ceiling, most of which were flecked with bits of grit and debris. In contrast, now there are great gobs of it, especially once you leave the windpipe and move out into the smaller air tubes.

There is so much mucus that as you pick your way down the many branching passageways, you must at times negotiate around obstructions or even force a path through the muck. As you go along down ever-smaller airway branchings, sometimes you have no choice about which way to go because the openings to some of them are completely blocked off with mucus. Others are just pinched shut for no apparent reason that you can see, but from your last trip, you realize that pressure on the outside of the tubes, from retained air in the lungs, can press on these small airways and choke them shut. From the ones that are still open you detect very little air flowing back at you.

Could all this mucus be the cause of the airway obstruction? Certainly the thick, gooey stuff must be part of the problem, because it surely makes it difficult for the air currents to get in and out. That is part of the explanation, but it looks to you as if there are other reasons as well, reasons which have nothing at all to do with the mucous debris in the air tube. You determine this because you notice some branchings that are wide open, not blocked at all with mucus, yet when you motor up to them to check things out, your airflow indicator detects barely a wisp of returning air from deeper in that part of the lung.

It is only when you reach the smallest airways that you see the main reason for the airflow problem. Down where the supporting scaffold of the cartilage arches and subsequent wall-stiffening plates of cartilage are no longer present, the air tube's walls are lax. This means that if the lung surrounding the bronchiole is overinflated because air cannot get out, it can push the tube shut. You have already seen a few examples of that. But you also see something else that is much more important.

This is the region where, on your last trip, you saw those bands of muscle tissue roping around the breathing tubes. Now you see that the diameters of all the small airways are a fraction of what they were before.

On your last trip it was a tight squeeze for you to get through; now you can barely make it farther, and you need to try several bronchioles before you can find one that has an opening you can even fit through. Once you make it inside at last you see the cause for this obstruction: the meshworks of muscle bands encircling the bronchioles have squeezed them shut like tiny rope nooses. Every single one of the bands is in spasm, which is why another word for an asthma attack is "bronchospasm." Why would your son's lungs do this? What possible use could there be for structures in the lung that squeeze off essential air? It seems crazy.

Our bodies do contain some structures that do not—as far as we know—do us any good and may cause us problems. You will read about one of these in the next chapter. But having the ability to pinch off bronchioles with these muscular bands, structures that function like hose clamps, does serve an important function. In an asthma attack they malfunction—in effect, they get confused—but, working properly, they do serve a useful function most of the time.

The lung's main job is to get oxygen into our bloodstream and get carbon dioxide out of it. To do this, nature has devised a clever way to bring a large volume of blood in very close proximity to the millions of tiny air sacs. On the microscopic scale you witnessed, this is all that is needed to accomplish the task—the laws of physics and chemistry will do the rest, with oxygen diffusing into the blood from the alveoli and carbon dioxide diffusing out of the blood and into the alveoli.

It is a wonderfully simple system, but it requires one important thing to work well: the blood and the air must be matched together efficiently. By that I mean it does no good if the blood rushes by alveolar units that do not have fresh air going in and out. Likewise, if there are places in the lung where only very meager blood flow reaches air sacs that are well ventilated, that air is wasted. When either of those things happens, air does not meet blood efficiently. Without those ropy, muscular bands on the bronchioles, such mismatching of blood and air would happen in much of the lung. Here is why.

The best explanation is to remember that liquid, like blood, sinks but air rises. Thus, when you are sitting upright in a chair, the air you breathe in wants to go to the upper parts of your lungs, but the blood flowing through your lungs tends to go toward their bottom. There is always some degree of this blood-air mismatch. To combat it, to match the air and the blood with each other, the lungs have two sets of regulators—one in the air tubes, one in the blood vessels.

The lung's blood vessels have the ability to constrict the diameter of some tiny branches and increase others. The effect is like the head gates of an irrigation system, directing more blood to one place than to another. The result is that more blood gets sent to the parts of the lung where the air is moving best.

The airway regulators are the ropy muscle bands around the bronchioles. When they contract, they pinch down on air tubes; when they relax, the tubes open up. This reflex allows the airway system to direct incoming air to those places where there is the best blood flow. The system is vital to how our bodies work. Unfortunately, the system can make mistakes. Asthma is an example of this; those little nooses around the small airways pull them closed when they should not. Moreover, they all pinch down at the same time, blocking the airways throughout the lung. Nature never intended that to happen.

Physiology lecture done, let us return to you and your vessel, squeezing your way through an inappropriately constricted air tube. When you finally make it through what is now a tiny bronchiole to reach an alveolar sac, you find this place has changed dramatically since your last visit, too. You now find yourself in a space twice the size of what it was when you were there last. The air is building up, trapped behind the constricted bronchioles, and overexpanding his lungs. It takes a huge amount of force to push any air out past all those tight, flow-restricting nooses. In fact, it is much more difficult to get the air out than it is to suck it in. Your son is doing the best he can, using all his chest muscles (remember the retractions in his upper chest), but he cannot get enough of the air out past the obstruction, so it backs up here. What can we do to help the situation? Anything?

When you and your son arrived in the emergency department, the staff quickly started several key treatments for asthma. The nurse immediately saw he was not getting enough oxygen into his blood, so she gave him some with an oxygen mask. On your trip down to his bronchioles you saw the reason for that need of extra oxygen; the bronchioles that are merely constricted by the muscle bands usually let through sufficient oxygen, but the ones blocked off, either by mucus or by the surrounding pressure, are useless for getting either oxygen into his system or carbon dioxide out. The oxygen mask helps by delivering extra oxygen to those air tubes that are still at least partly open. It buys time for the other medicines to work.

Along with the oxygen, the emergency department staff gave him a medicine that goes right after one of the root problems, the constriction of the bronchioles. A medicine called albuterol (one of several that work in the same way) specifically relaxes all those constricted muscle bands, those little nooses squeezing shut the bronchioles and pinching off his airways. You already had given him some at home, but the emergency department can give much higher and more frequent doses safely, something you cannot do yourself. As you turn your vessel around to begin your journey back from his air sacs you can already see things improving—those pernicious bands of spasmodic muscles are already relaxing, releasing their grip on his small airways.

The medicine causing this improvement is misting all around you as you travel back. It works fast. When your son breathes it in as a fine mist, it soaks into the walls of the air tubes and passes through to the muscle bands, on which it has an immediate relaxing effect. The muscle cords loosen, and the tiny passageways begin to return to their normal size. For some children, this can take some time, often a day or more of treatment, sometimes several, to get all the airways open. But albuterol and drugs like it are very effective at accomplishing this.

So the airway constriction is soon better. But what about all that mucus you encountered in the airway? Where did it come from, why is it there, and what can be done about it? It clearly was part of the problem, too. The answer is that there is more to asthma than just constriction of the bronchioles. If that were all there was to it, drugs like albuterol would solve you son's problem fairly quickly.

As you have seen, in asthma the bronchioles constrict when they should not, and they do it everywhere in the lung, compounding the problem. The lung activates a normally important and useful reflex but at the wrong time and in the wrong places. All the mucus you saw in the airways is evidence of another deranged phenomenon.

Besides airway constriction, the hallmark of asthma is inflammation around the airways. You saw inflammation at work in chapter 1, how it is a complicated and well-coordinated cascade of events: the tissues send out a call for help in the form of chemical messages, various specialized cells like phagocytes hear the call, rush to the scene, and go to work. The substances phagocytes and similar cells use to do their work, things they release at the scene, are powerful weapons. Although they can destroy germs, they also can damage the surrounding cells. The more inflammatory cells present, the greater the potential damage from such friendly fire.

The inflammation around an asthmatic's airway is—like the constricted bronchioles—a useful body system gone awry; it is in this situation harming rather than helping. The inflammatory fires not only do no good, they worsen the problem by contributing to the blockage of airflow. The trigger for this inappropriate inflammation is probably the same as the trigger that brought on the airway constriction, such as a viral respiratory illness or something in the environment—pollen, for example.

Doctors treat asthma by targeting both the airway constriction and the inflammation. Albuterol and drugs like it target the constriction. We usually use a class of drugs called steroids—inhaled, taken by mouth, or injected into the vein—to dampen the inflammation. In addition, we have drugs that block mucous production, as well as others that reduce the effects of the chemical signals that drive inflammation.

A child's body is a magnificent thing to watch in action, especially from the inside, at the cellular level. Most of the time we doctors assume the body knows what it is doing because it is smarter than we are regarding its own needs. But sometimes this is not so—the body is sometimes confused and turns its own protective systems back on itself. The phenomenon of asthma is one of those times. Fortunately, as you have seen, we have ways of correcting this and nudging a child's lungs back toward their proper function.

In your son's case, inhaled albuterol and steroids, plus some oral steroids for a few days do the trick. Within a day he is back to his normal self and feeling fine. In the future, though, he should probably take some of his asthma medication before he goes to the zoo.

· *4* ·

Not All Body Parts Are Useful:
A Look Inside a Sick Appendix

We generally assume that every part of our body has a useful function, even if we are not precisely sure what that function is. The history of medicine has more than a few examples in which the importance of a particular organ was unknown for centuries until medical science finally figured out what it was for. Because of that we should be careful about concluding that any body part is useless and worthy of being discarded. It is a good general principle to follow. But in spite of that principle, there are some parts of us that really do appear to have no current purpose.

The tailbone, or coccyx, is an example of what is called a vestigial organ—one that links humankind to our distant past, when our ancestors apparently had tails. Ear muscles may be an example of the same thing. Acute hearing, for a creature in the wild, can spell the difference between finding dinner and becoming someone else's dinner. Most mammals can move their ears around, even swivel them completely about, allowing for focusing of sound and sharper hearing. Doing this requires muscles in the ears. Humans generally do not have these muscles anymore, although a few of us can wiggle our ears, indicating the old system still works, if only a little.

Generally these curiosities from our ancient past are no more than that—curiosities. Sometimes, however, the past comes back to bite us. This chapter takes you on a pair of explorations to see what can happen then.

Imagine your six-year-old daughter has been ill since perhaps the day before yesterday—it is a little hard for you to tell because it seemed to come on gradually. It was also difficult to say just where her problem lay, at least at first. But today her discomfort seems pretty clearly to be with her stomach. When you go into her room in the morning you find she has not gotten up for school, something unusual for her. She says her tummy hurts. You press on it a bit and find that it does seem to bother her when you push down. When you put your hand on her forehead it feels hot, and a thermometer confirms she has a fever. She has no appetite at all and says she feels like throwing up. With your encouragement, she does drink a little juice but soon afterward vomits.

Her older sister was ill last week with several days of mild fever and vomiting, and you think your younger daughter probably has a similar case of stomach flu. But her sister did not have the same kind of pain—in her it was more of a vague ache. Concerned, you decide to take her to the doctor. It is probably just the flu, but it seems best to be sure.

What might be going on inside her? As with the previous scenarios, understanding what is wrong now requires some understanding of what the world inside a child's gastrointestinal tract normally looks like. So before you learn what the problem is now, you should first cast yourself back a few days and explore the area when she was well, traveling inside the same miniature vessel that took you to the ear and the lung. On the last chapter's trip your craft was primarily an aerial hovercraft, since the lungs are mostly all about air. This trip requires its submarine capabilities, since the world of the digestive tract, the stomach and intestines, is primarily liquid.

The digestive tract is really nothing more than a long tube, beginning at the mouth and ending at the rectum. Although we think of it as being inside us, in a very real sense it is not—it is actually outside us. I say this because it connects with the outside world directly on both ends, so something traveling all the way through never really penetrates the body's interior.

On a global level the process of digestion is simple. It consists of passing what we eat along the tube, meanwhile chemically altering and refining the stuff as it moves along, taking into our bodies what we want, and letting the remainder pass on through. The long mouth-to-rectum tube has a series of discrete locations in it; think of it as a bunch of caves connected to each other by a continuous tunnel.

The first room is the mouth, so you start your trip there, first traveling over the surface of your daughter's tongue until you get to the base of it in the back of her throat. So far the road to the intestinal tract is the same as the road to the lung. Below you sits the epiglottis, the flap of tissue that guards the entryway to the lungs. As you learned last chapter, it is vigilant about keeping things out of the lungs that do not belong there. Getting to the gateway to the stomach is much easier than negotiating the portal beneath the epiglottis. In fact, the route down to the stomach is generally the default pathway for anything that comes in through the mouth.

You pass over your daughter's epiglottis and proceed on to the back of her throat. There you dive down into the pink tube leading to the stomach, called the esophagus. The walls of the esophagus are muscles, and they immediately close in all around you. In the clutches of these strong muscles, you are unable to move at all. Unless something changes, you are not going anywhere, and it will be a short trip.

In a moment, though, something does change. You start to move, and you realize it is because the muscles of the esophagus themselves are propelling you onward. They do this by relaxing just in front of you and squeezing together just behind you, moving you along like fingers squeezing a tube of toothpaste. You try to look outside your window, but you cannot see anything because the tissue outside is wrapped tightly around your craft.

It takes a little while for you to travel down the full length of the esophagus and reach the stomach. This is because when we swallow it takes a few seconds for the waves of the muscular contractions in the esophagus to propel whatever is in our mouths into our stomachs. Swallowing is something we do frequently, every minute or so. Our salivary glands, located in our cheeks and on the floor of our mouths under our tongues, are continually producing saliva and dripping it into our mouths. This needs to be swallowed. You were stuck at the top of the esophagus until your daughter made one of these periodic swallows to shove you along.

You ride the esophageal muscle wave like a surfer until it shoots you out into the stomach. For a moment you find yourself flying through the air, then splash down into a lake of dark fluid, mixed with assorted large chunks of your daughter's macaroni and cheese lunch. When you bob to the surface and look outside you find you are in a tanklike cavity. An adult's stomach holds about three quarts, a child's proportionately less.

You shine your light overhead and see a ceiling and pink walls with deep folds in them. There is liquid running down the walls everywhere into the pool, steadily raising the fluid level, until it suddenly drops at intervals with a gurgling sound.

Although fresh liquid is constantly weeping from the walls and ceiling, most of the fluid in our stomachs comes from what we drink. You can easily tell this is the case with your daughter from the bright raspberry hue of the lake, the same color as the fruit punch she drank an hour ago. The lake itself is far from a quiet lagoon. Besides the occasional gurgles when the level drops, it is also a seething, churning place, with bubbles and whirlpools everywhere.

What you are seeing are the opening stages of digestion at work. Digestion actually begins in our mouths, since saliva has substances in it, called enzymes, that begin to break down food into its simple chemical forms, but it is in the stomach where the process really gets rolling. And rolling is the right word, because the stomach turns and mashes the food all around like a blender, mechanically mixing it all together. Central to this process is mixing and folding gastric juice, the stuff you see dripping off the walls, into the brew.

Gastric juice is strong stuff. It contains additional enzymes to those in saliva, especially ones that break down protein such as meat. Gastric juice also contains acid—strong acid. The acid is so strong that when it gets out of the stomach, such as when a little splashes back up into the esophagus, it hurts. That is heartburn, although you may hear it called the fancier, descriptive term gastro-esophageal reflux. The stomach itself has a special lining that protects it from all the acid and enzymes. This protection can fail sometimes; when it does, the person can get an ulcer. Fortunately for you, the outer covering of your vessel is impervious to gastric juice, otherwise you might get digested yourself.

You soon notice something else about the place—the noise, above and beyond those occasional gurgles. On your trip to the lungs you became accustomed to the back-and-forth whoosh of air. You also easily heard the lub-dub of your son's heart when you passed it by. What you hear now is completely different. It is much louder, and more than a little eerie sounding. You hear, seemingly at random intervals, both high-pitched wails and squeaks and low bass rumbles. Digestion is certainly a noisy process. Often we can hear stomachs growl from several feet away.

Hearing a heartbeat requires a stethoscope; hearing digestion often requires nothing special at all.

The noise primarily comes from air moving through our systems, air we swallow either along with food or all by itself. A good part of a carbonated beverage ends up inside us as the gas carbon dioxide. As you found, the esophagus closes tightly around what it is swallowing, but it is impossible to avoid swallowing at least a little air, and most of the time the stomach is a mixture of liquid and air. The air can either move along the system or be burped back out, something children seem to love to do.

You dive beneath the churning surface and motor onward. The turbulence is such that you feel as if you are navigating the swirling waters at the base of a huge waterfall. By the time you reach the lower part of the stomach you see that the material you are in is now all liquid—the chunks are gone, although it is still a thick liquid. It does not take the stomach long to liquefy all that macaroni.

You soon find yourself at the lower outlet from the stomach. It looks like the valve to a pipe, and that is exactly what it is. The valve is called the pylorus, and it opens now and then to drain a portion of the stomach's contents. It is a key control point for the digestive system. The stomach can store a lot of food, but our digestive system would get overwhelmed if it all rushed out of the stomach at once after a large meal.

The pylorus keeps a steady and manageable amount of food moving further on down. When the lower reaches of the intestines are ready for more, the valve opens. Otherwise it stays shut, waiting for the proper time to let more through. If the pylorus malfunctions, two sorts of problems can result. If the valve is too small or fails to operate properly, a person can get a blockage of that flow, and things back up into the stomach. This is occasionally seen in small infants, especially boys, who can have a pylorus that is too muscular and tight, a condition called pyloric stenosis. (It is easily fixed with simple surgery.) In contrast, if the pylorus is always wide open or gone entirely, such as from previous surgery, a person can get too much food dumping through too fast, and the digestive system cannot handle the flood.

Like a boat waiting its turn at a set of locks, you wait for the pylorus to open. When it does, you ride along with the next surge of food. That food is already being digested and broken down into its component parts, both by the mechanical mixing in the stomach and by the acid and the stomach enzymes. More, and different, enzymes get added to the food as you move downstream.

Once through the pylorus you find yourself in the small intestine. It is called small because of its diameter, not its length, which is actually quite long. The length of the small intestine varies from person to person, but it is usually about twenty feet long in an adult, proportionately less in a child. This means that it needs to be coiled in our bellies in order for it to fit inside us.

The very first part of the small intestine, called the duodenum, does not move around; it is fixed in one place by the tissues surrounding it. It crosses over our backbones just below our stomachs. Unlike the duodenum, the rest of the intestines, large and small, are not stuck in one place in the abdomen. They move around, something that you can feel happening in yourself from time to time if you pay attention. It is easy to understand why they need to move. The intestines need to accommodate a stream of air and liquid that varies greatly throughout the day. They need to expand, contract, and squeeze everything along, something they could not do very well if they were restricted.

In the duodenum there is not much need to use your engines, except to maneuver back and forth a little; you simply go with the flow. As you come around a corner you look up in your searchlight beam and see a pipe in the ceiling squirting green liquid into the stream. This pipe is called the common duct. It leads back to two essential digestive organs—the liver and the pancreas. There are separate, smaller pipes from each of these organs that join together just before it spills out its contents into the intestine. The green stuff you see coming out of the pipe is a mixture of bile from the liver and juice from the pancreas. These materials are needed for proper digestion of fats and proteins.

Rounding another corner, you leave the duodenum and slide into the next part of the intestine, called the jejunum. Digestion from bile and the brew of all the enzymes continues here. In fact, it is the place where most of the digested material gets absorbed into our systems. You shine your light on the wall. It is yellow pink in color, has a soft, corrugated surface, and surrounds you with a series of concentric folds in its surface. That surface is key to digestion; all along it are tiny projecting fingers of tissue, like feathers, that have still more enzymes on them that are essential for digestion of carbohydrates—sugar and starches, such as pasta or potatoes. They also have special systems for absorbing amino acids, the building blocks of proteins, as well as ones to take in the fats and oils we eat.

The jejunum is filled with a rich soup. As the process of digestion makes it more molecularly simple, the cells lining the tube actively pump it into the body's circulation. As you drift along, you notice that the soup is getting thinner and easier to see through and that the tunnel is just a little narrower. You are now in what is called the ileum, the lower part of the small intestine. By now your daughter has absorbed most of the nutrients of her lunch into her body, but the little that remains can be grabbed by the ileum. The main job of the ileum, besides absorbing what gets missed further upstream, is to absorb specific vitamins and iron, as well as recycling the bile that came from the liver so it can be used for another round of digestion. By the time you reach the end of the ileum, nearly all the nutrients are gone, leaving largely indigestible things like plant fiber floating in the residual water.

As you maneuver down this intestinal tunnel you hardly need your craft's engine at all. A powerful current carries you on your way. That current is not steady, however; it comes in rushes of movement every several minutes or so that lurch you along. When you look out your rear window you see how those waves of movement happen. Every so often the entire cavity—walls, ceiling, floor—collapses together and squeezes the intestinal contents along. It comes from rhythmic contractions of muscles in the intestines. We normally easily feel this in ourselves, especially after we eat. The contractions move down the intestines in stately, controlled waves, much like those you see when you slowly shake a long garden hose laid out on the ground.

The further you travel, the more you notice something else—germs. As soon as you left the stomach, you began to see bacteria. There were even a few living in the stomach, although they need to be hardy indeed to survive in that harsh environment. We swallow bacteria with everything we eat, since food is not completely sterile, even though we wash and clean it to remove the mass of bacteria. These germs pass through the stomach to the small intestine, just as you did. Once in the intestine, it is not surprising that bacteria thrive there—the partially digested food is a banquet table for them. Their numbers steadily increase all the way down the intestine.

By the time you reach the ileum, there are huge numbers of bacteria all around you. When you investigated your son's ear infection, you saw bacteria then, too, but nothing like this. For one thing, there are many different kinds of bacteria here. For another, they look to be millions of times more numerous than they did even in his badly infected ear. It is a city of germs. You flash your light at the walls, expecting with all these germs to see the kind of bacteria-inflamed tissue you saw in your son's infected ear or his finger, but here the bacteria seem to be causing no irritation, no problems at all. In fact, intestinal bacteria even help us by manufacturing a needed vitamin, vitamin K, which we cannot make ourselves. The germs of a digestive tube and the tube's owner cohabit with one another just fine. How can this be?

The reason we can handle so many germs in our intestines is that we have there an extremely effective defense system. The most important component of this system is a kind of local immunity similar to what you saw in your son's ear. The intestinal wall protects itself quite well through a combination of mucous coating and specialized cells that live there, which release germ-fighting substances. The intestines also have back-up systems if a few of the germs should break through the initial barriers. In spite of these defenses, the relationship between us and the germs within our intestines is always a little tense; a serious breakdown in the intestinal wall can upset the balance and send the germs streaming into our bloodstream to spread throughout the body.

Meanwhile, back in the ileum, you shine your light ahead and see your pathway is coming to an abrupt end in a blind pouch. When you get closer and can see a little better, you notice there is a way out of the end of the ileum. There is what appears to be a round porthole there. It looks a little like the pylorus, the valve out of the stomach, only smaller. It is indeed another valve, called the ileocecal valve. It is the connection between the small intestine and the large intestine. It opens and you zip through, leaving the small intestine for the large intestine, also called the colon.

Compared with the small intestine, the large intestine looks, well, large—it is at least several times the diameter of the tube you just left. In an adult, it is three to four feet long and several inches in diameter. What you really notice, though, are the germs. Here the numbers of bacteria are enormously increased, hundreds of times over, beyond what you saw in the lower portions of the small intestine. The fluid in the end of the ileum was also much cleaner than the stuff in this place.

Disoriented in the murk, since even your light has trouble in this mess, you make a wrong turn. Instead of going left, where the lazy stream of liquid is heading, you first travel to the rightward and downward, but you soon realize this is a blind alley. It is called the cecum, and it is indeed a blind alley, created because the ileum does not join the colon at its end, but rather at the side of the colon a bit up from the end. At the very end of the cecum you dimly see a very small opening through the gloom. You doubt it leads anywhere, but you are curious, so you navigate to it and briefly go inside. Once inside, you find you were correct—it does not go anywhere. It is itself a smaller blind alley, an inch or so in length, at the end of the larger blind alley of the cecum. It is the appendix.

Turning your now very dirty vessel about, you travel quickly back out the appendix, across the cecum, and past the ileocecal valve, the place you entered the large intestine. You continue on down the tunnel, noting as you go that the soup is getting drier and thicker. Indeed, the main job of the large intestine is to absorb water back into the body. Finally you exit the digestive tube, your journey of discovery completed. After giving your craft a good wash down, you are ready to start over, this time to understand what may be the cause of your daughter's belly pain and fever.

The first part of your return journey, down her esophagus and into her stomach, looks superficially similar to what you saw before, but there are some subtle hints that everything is not right. You notice your daughter's tongue and cheeks are not the same healthy pink they were on your first trip. Now her tongue is coated with a bit of grayish crust, and the sides of her mouth do not appear to be as moist.

These things are what one sees inside the mouth of a child who is mildly dehydrated, a little dry, as doctors say. The dehydration comes from not drinking much, vomiting, and fever. All of us, especially children, have a more or less fixed, obligatory water loss each hour.

One source for this is urine. We have a certain minimal amount of urine our kidneys must make each hour to stay functional. Both adults and children have the ability to urinate less when necessary, conserving water that way, but a child's kidneys are less able to do this than are an adult's. Thus, some of your daughter's dehydration comes from her obligatory water loss in urine. We also lose water through breathing. This is because our exhaled breath is completely saturated with water—its relative humidity is 100 percent. You can see this when you breathe on a mirror and it fogs up. Thus, simple breathing takes water from a child's body. A third cause of your child's mild dehydration is her fever. As a rough rule of thumb, water loss increases about 10 percent over baseline for each degree of fever.

Once in her stomach, you notice not much is there, just a puddle of gastric juice, barely enough to keep your vessel afloat. Compared with your first trip, things are also very, very quiet—too quiet. You hear the occasional noise, but overall her intestinal tract is strangely still. When you do hear a noise, it is not the low-pitched growl you recall. Instead, it sounds like a high-pitched squeak.

When you pass through her pylorus and out of her stomach you notice a few other things. The first is that you need to use your motors to propel yourself, unlike your last trip. Then your craft barely needed its own engine, because it was pushed steadily along in the stream by the muscular waves that squeezed the intestine every few minutes. Now those rhythmic contractions are gone—the whole river is stagnant and still. Since she has not been eating much, there is little food material there. It is mostly a mixture of bile and gastric and pancreatic juices. You do not see much there in the way of nutrition.

The stagnant pools explain why she vomited: everything has simply backed up in the small intestine. Normally our digestive system continues to produce liquid, such as gastric juice and saliva, even between meals, and there is always some swallowed air. This mixture needs to move along because more is arriving behind it. When nothing moves in the small intestine, we vomit because there is no place for the stomach contents to go. Our stomach rumblings in this abnormal situation greatly decrease or disappear, as your daughter's have. Often, what a child throws up in this situation is stained green from bile, since bile often backs up from the duodenum, backward through the pylorus, and into the stomach. Understandably, in these circumstances a child loses her appetite, and your daughter has eaten little in the past twenty-four hours.

The condition of nothing moving at all in the intestinal tract is called an ileus. There are many disorders of the intestines that can cause this to happen. If it becomes severe, we treat it with a mechanical solution, since it is a mechanical problem. What we do is slide a long tube, called a naso-gastric tube, through the nose and down into the stomach and then hook the outside of the tube to a suction device. Once in place, they often have to stay in for a day or two. It is unpleasant to have one of these tubes, of course, although the natural tendency a child feels to gag when the tube first touches the back of her throat generally passes soon. In spite of the mild discomfort a nasogastric tube causes, they do make a child with a severe ileus feel better. They stem the nausea and vomiting, because they suck out the air and digestive juices that are backing up and causing the unpleasant symptoms.

So your child has an ileus. That fact does not explain everything that is going on, but it does explain at least a few of her symptoms. It also confirms there is something abnormal going on deeper in her digestive system to cause the abnormal stoppage of transport through the system. To find out exactly what this something is you need to get further inside. So, putting your craft in gear, you journey on.

On your last trip you rode a river. Now at times your vehicle must become an all-terrain vehicle, crawling from pool to pool of stagnant fluid. Before you have gone much further, you start to see more fluid again—that is encouraging. But the fluid is not a steady river, like before. Now her small intestine appears to be a series of caves with a deep, isolated lake at the bottom of each one. You find yourself passing periodically through high-ceilinged caverns, so high that your light barely shows what is at the top of them. Her entire small intestine now consists of a series of large collections of air up above and stagnant pools below. The chambers alternate with hairpin turns of the intestinal tunnel that force you to dive your craft down underwater before surfacing again in the next cavern.

The landscape you are traveling through is very typical for an ileus, seen from the inside. The way we usually see it from the outside is with an x-ray, on which it has a very characteristic appearance. If we take an x-ray of the person's abdomen with them sitting up all those caverns look like a series of hairpins on the x-ray. Each has its own pocket of air and a lake of fluid below. Listening to a child's belly with a stethoscope when there is an ileus also produces characteristic findings; instead of the usual occasional rumbles, one hears long periods of silence with perhaps only a very occasional high-pitched squeak.

After sloshing through a succession of these air-fluid pockets, you finally reach the ileocecal valve at the end. You pop through the valve and find yourself again in the large intestine. Once again, nothing is the same.

The first thing you notice is that things are strangely quiet, as in the small intestine. Nothing is moving anywhere, and although there are still millions more bacteria here than there were on the upstream side of the ileocecal valve, it is much less murky than before, giving you a better view of the walls around you. When you shine your light to the right, down toward the cecum, you see those walls are slightly reddened. At the end of the cecum, where the opening to the appendix is, the rim of colon wall around the opening is bright red. The area is also a little swollen, obscuring the fine detail of the surface. You think surely that must be where the root of your daughter's trouble lies, so you motor down to her appendix to investigate.

You find the opening completely blocked off, sealed up tight. You have been there before and know the doorway is not deep, and you are determined to get inside because you are convinced that is where the trouble lies. So by backing up a distance and taking a good run at the opening, you succeed in forcing your way inside.

You immediately find yourself floating in precisely the same kind of soup you last encountered in your son's middle ear when he had an infection there. Bacteria are everywhere, and so are phagocytes. As in the ear, many of the phagocytes are bloated, stuffed chock-full of bacteria. Others are so full they ruptured open, spilling fragments of dead and dying bacteria back into the mix.

Although the scene resembles an infected middle ear in some ways, in other ways it differs. One obvious difference is that in the ear the invading bacteria were all of the same type. This is because they were all relatives. They were all direct offspring of the first pioneering germs to reach the middle ear, set up shop there, and begin reproducing rapidly. In the cavity of the appendix it is different. There are all manner of bacteria here—long rod-shaped ones, short stubby ones, and spherical ones. This is because they are representative of all the varied bacteria that live just outside in the colon.

Shining your light around the inside of the appendix shows you it is now twice the size it was last time, because the pressure building up inside it has stretched the walls. The walls themselves are bright red. This is partly because the tissues are inflamed and angry. But they are also red because there is a little blood oozing from the walls and running down around you. No wonder your daughter has worsening abdominal pain—you feel some sympathetic pain yourself just looking at these swollen and tender tissues. She has appendicitis, and appendicitis hurts.

All around you there is cellular debris, making navigation difficult, but you want to go just a little bit farther to see if you can discover more about what is causing all this trouble. Finally you reach the end of the line, the furthest reaches of the appendix. The wall there looks very unusual. There are multiple blotchy, purplish-black areas scattered across the surface. These are set in areas surrounded by intensely red rings of tissue. When you look closely at the largest of these blotches, you see nothing but total blackness. Coming closer still, you shine your light directly at the spot, and the beam disappears into the blackness beyond. It is, you discover, not the appendix wall at all. There is a gaping, ragged hole at the end of the appendix that opens out into whatever is beyond. Your daughter not only has appendicitis, but the swollen appendix has burst from the pressure inside.

What is out there in the black beyond is what we call the peritoneal cavity, the name for the space inside the belly that holds the stomach, intestines, liver, and spleen. Having come this far, you decide to investigate even further. You drive out through the hole. What you find there is a different world; now you are truly within the body itself, in a place which, unlike the lungs, ear, or intestines, does not normally connect to anything on the outside in any way. It is normally a closed, sealed-up space.

You cruise upward to get some elevation, the better to look down on the appendix and the hole in its end. Glancing around, you realize now you are looking at the other side of her intestines. Her small intestine lies beneath you in convoluted loops; her large intestine drapes from side to side across her lower abdomen. You can see the appendix, swollen like a fat, red sausage, hanging off the end of the cecum. From this vantage point, you can also see that the glistening membrane that lines this entire space, called the peritoneum, is red and sore looking around near the hole in the appendix. This, in turn, has made the overlying wall of her abdomen sore, which is why it hurt when you pushed on it.

Next you glide down to the area around the hole in the appendix. What you find there are more phagocytes, so many that there are mounds and mounds of them. They are surrounded by germs. Unlike what you saw in your trips to the ear and the finger, here the germs definitely have the upper hand. There are just so many of them that they overwhelm the fresh musters of phagocytes as soon as they arrive. The germs are doing so well because the enormous concentration of them in the colon gave them an immense head start on your daughter's defenses. Once they have broken through the appendix wall, there is no stopping them.

Now you have seen all you need to see and have all the information you need to have. It is time to speed back to your daughter's side and take care of her problem. As you travel back, here is some information about appendicitis to consider as you go.

A common ailment, particularly among children, appendicitis happens when the opening of the appendix becomes blocked for some reason. Such blockage can occur from bits of stool getting caught there or from swelling of the tissues around the appendix. Swelling sufficient to close it off can happen following a mild intestinal infection. It is very like the scenario in chapter 2, when swelling around the auditory tube in the nasal cavity blocked it off and caused ear infection behind. Having its proper drainage obstructed often leads to trouble for the appendix, too—infection behind the blockage. The appendix is at a disadvantage compared with the ear and the lung because the area is already teeming with germs.

In spite of the known association of obstruction of the opening with subsequent appendicitis, some patients are just like your daughter—in them, as with her, there is nothing obvious that might be closing off the opening. It just seems to swell shut on its own. Once it does, though, events proceed in the same way in all cases.

As the swelling gets worse, the pressure inside the appendix rises. At a certain point, the pressure is enough to press shut the network of blood vessels in the surrounding walls. This puts the team of local immunity players at a tremendous disadvantage, because they rely on the bloodstream to bring supplies and reinforcements. Without that help, plus the fact that hordes of bacteria are already poised and ready, the rapidly dividing bacteria begin to win the battle, and their penetration into the walls causes even more swelling. It is an axiom of medicine that inflamed tissues without good blood flow cannot survive for long under bacterial attack—they are like an army surrounded and cut off from its supply lines. The appendiceal wall softens and then ultimately gives way. You saw the results.

Your daughter's symptoms followed the usual pattern for appendicitis. First came the stoppage of normal intestinal activity, with its nausea, loss of appetite, and vomiting. As her appendix became more inflamed, she developed steadily worsening pain over the lower right part of her abdomen and a fever. Now that you know all that, what do we do for your daughter?

Appendicitis nearly always requires surgery to remove the appendix, along with any infected pus and tissue that may be surrounding it. It is an extremely common operation in children because appendicitis is an extremely common problem. Until some years ago, surgery meant that the surgeon made an incision in the lower right part of a child's abdomen over the appendix and removed it.

These days, the majority of simple appendectomies are done using a device called a laparoscope, a lighted tube the surgeon can look through. The surgeon makes several small incisions in the abdomen; one of these is to put the laparoscope through, the others are for other instruments. Using this technique, the surgeon can look at the appendix while he grasps it with one of his instruments, cuts it from the end of the cecum, seals off the stump of where the appendix was, so no more bacteria can get through, and pulls the instruments back out.

In comparison with the open technique, children who have laparoscopic appendectomies usually recover from the surgery faster and go home sooner. Not all cases can be done this way, however, because the particular circumstances and extent of the inflammatory process vary from child to child. Your own daughter's doctor immediately recognized her symptoms for what they were, called a surgeon, and within a few hours later, your daughter was resting comfortably in a hospital bed. A few days later she was completely fine.

The inflammation in the tissues around her appendix plays out the same way it did in chapter 1, the infected finger, and heals in just the same way. The inflamed appendix is driving the process, so once it is removed, there is no further fuel for the inflammatory flames. Now the same clean-up crew you saw in the finger can move in and do their job. They clear away all the cellular debris and lay down new blood capillaries as needed. They mop up any stray bacteria that are still in the tissues, once again confining the germs to where they belong—out in the tunnel of the large intestine. As with the inflamed, infected finger you saw, most doctors give a child with a ruptured appendix some antibiotics to help things along after surgery, but the main treatment is removing the inflamed appendix.

Your daughter now has a few small incisions that need healing. These do so quickly, because there are no bacteria in the area and the inflammation is minimal. The same fibroblasts of the sort you saw at work in the finger wake up, replicate themselves into many more fibroblasts, and draw together the edges of the incision. The fibroblasts do leave their calling card once healing is done, which is the visible scar in the skin.

Many people go through life with their appendix causing them no trouble, but for many others, it is an organ that gives nothing but trouble. As far as we can tell, the appendix does not help us in any way, at least these days. Millennia ago the appendix might have served a useful purpose. We surmise this because animals who are grazing herbivores, such as horses, have an immense appendix; it is nearly as large as their colon. For them, it appears to be an important organ of digestion. Perhaps when our ancient ancestors ate more rough plants, as horses do now, their appendixes served them well by allowing them to digest vegetation we can no longer eat. That is an interesting thing to speculate about, but we do not know for certain if it is true.

· 5 ·

How We Know the Enemy:
A Close-up View of the Immune System

Several of the previous chapters have taken a military tone. Germs attack a child's body. The phagocytes, aided by a variety of other troops and materials, fight back. The result of this struggle is a messy battlefield littered with casualties. The cellular reconstruction crew then carts away the debris, buries the dead, and rebuilds the damage caused by the battle. It is a fanciful but still useful way to think of things. Yet up until now we have passed over a key aspect of the body's defense mechanisms: How does a child's body know who the enemy is? How does the intelligence-gathering division of our defense system work, identifying who and what needs to be attacked? Most importantly, what keeps us from using all these sophisticated weapons against ourselves?

This chapter is about how these things happen. It is about the immune system. Immunology is among the most complicated and difficult to understand (and difficult to explain) subjects in all of medicine. But if you are to understand how your child heals, you need to learn something about it. Complicated or not, anyone can learn enough to do that.

The fundamental problem faced by all the body's defenses, the immune system included, is distinguishing friend from foe, self from nonself. Our bodies are made up of billions of tiny cells, nearly all of which are organized into specialized teams to do specialized work. You have already seen many examples of this, and the level of cellular specialization is quite astonishing. Even when we look at an individual organ, such as our liver, we find that within that organ, there is division of labor among the cells who do different varieties of things. Rarely can one kind of cell do the work of another kind.

The paradox is that, even within this vast, complex system of specialized cells, there is one thing that unites them all, a common similarity—they are all part of the same individual's body. In other words, my cells are not your cells. Even if a specialized cell in my liver is doing the exact same work as the equivalent highly specialized cell in your liver, my cell is still different from yours in a fundamental way—it is on my body's team and not yours. If a surgeon were to put one of your cells inside of me (assuming we are not identical twins), my body would attack it. The only way to prevent that from happening is to manipulate my immune system so it is confused about what is me and what is you, what is self and what is non-self.

As with earlier chapters, we begin with a journey, although this one will be different from the previous ones because it will require more time. You will need to live inside your trusty exploration vehicle for a few days at least as you watch things unfold. Since you will be gone so long, we will not use the example of one of your own children but one of a friend. Your friend can look after yours while you are gone exploring.

Your friend is taking her son to the doctor for a routine vaccination, something that will protect him from getting a specific infectious illness. Although many childhood vaccines are mixtures of several things, each component of the mix is specific for one thing. We mix them together mostly for convenience and to reduce the number of shots a child needs.

The vaccine your friend's child is getting this morning is against a bacterium with the scientific name of *Hemophilus influenzae*, or H. flu for short. H. flu has nothing to do with true influenza, the flu virus, even though researchers thought it did when they named it nearly a century ago. Until we had this vaccine, H. flu was a frequent cause of serious, even fatal illness in small children. It often infected the lungs and the airway, but its most serious target was a child's brain. The vaccine has led to a dramatic drop in cases, although we still see one from time to time in an unvaccinated child.

Imagine you have packed your vessel full of supplies for a long expedition, including plenty to read, because there will be some intervals when nothing exciting happens. You begin your trip inside the vaccine syringe the nurse is about to inject into the leg of your friend's child. She first wipes his skin with a pad of alcohol to kill any skin bacteria that might use the opportunity to crawl in and cause trouble at the needle puncture site. Then she pokes the needle in, pushes the plunger, and you are off.

You first find yourself inside a pocket in his leg muscle formed by the liquid that came in through the needle. Over the next few hours that pocket collapses as the liquid seeps into the surrounding tissue, although you can still see ample amounts of it around your craft. You gaze out the window, awaiting developments, but nothing is happening. After several hours of fruitless watching you give up and go back to the vessel's living quarters to have dinner and sleep until tomorrow. Perhaps something interesting will turn up then.

The next morning you look out to see that the tissue surrounding you is unchanged. You are lodged among a series of parallel, red muscle fibers. They are supplied by the sort of blood capillary meshwork you are now used to seeing; red blood cells march past, unloading the oxygen the muscle needs to do its work. You amuse yourself by watching the muscle fibers contract and relax as your friend's son uses his legs to run around.

Finally, your patience is rewarded. Out the windows you see some amoeba-like cells steadily crawling your way. They look quite a bit like the neutrophils-turned-phagocytes you have seen before, but there are differences. These cells look calmer, more deliberate in their actions, and they do not have the full load of dark granules you saw in the germ-fighting phagocytes. Before too much longer, you are surrounded by them. Who are they, and what are they doing?

The cells are called macrophages, and you have seen them before. Some of them were involved in the cleanup of the infected finger in chapter 1. Today they have another job, although it is really related to their mundane cleanup duties. They have again come to scavenge the debris, in this case the injected vaccine material, and haul it off, like any other cellular junk. But they have also come to snoop around and to investigate just what you are and what your business is.

Macrophages are members of a whole family of important cells that constitute the first responders of the immune system. They live throughout the body, like the scattered sentinels of an early warning system, but there is a particularly large number of them beneath the skin. This makes sense, since a common site of germ invasion is a break in the skin. As soon as they arrive, they begin scooping up the vaccine material with which you arrived. A few of them even crawl over your vessel, clearly suspicious of your intentions.

The H. flu vaccine, like most vaccines, is made artificially in a laboratory from material that mimics the material found on the surface of the germ. Some vaccines use pieces of the actual germ—killed first, of course. But since researchers long ago identified precisely what on the H. flu surface is needed to stimulate protective immunity in children, the vaccine contains only that part.

The macrophages draw the vaccine material inside themselves, chop it up, and move it back to their surface. They do this so other cells can see it. But they do not just randomly put it on their surface—they connect it with a cellular message, a signal to other cells that says something like this: "See this? It's not one of us—it's a foreign enemy." Not every kind of cell can interpret the message. The ones that can are part of the immune system. After the macrophages have cleaned up the vaccine, they wander off. Macrophages have powerful tools for dismantling debris, but fortunately your vessel is equipped with sufficient stealth technology that, after sniffing over your surface a bit, they leave you alone. You turn on your engines to follow them to see where they are going, glad that the waiting is over.

Where they are going is to a nearby outpost for the immune system, a lymph node. These structures are found throughout the body. They are the lumps you feel in the front of your neck, in the crease of your groin, or high up in your armpit. They are strategically positioned to collect the macrophages wandering throughout the tissues of the body. An extensive spiderweb of thin canals forms an easy path for the macrophages to travel to them. Lymph nodes are crucial for fighting infections. This is why you feel them swell if there is infection in the area, such as the nodes in your neck with a sore throat or tenderness in your groin crease if you have an infection on your toe, like a blister.

When the macrophages reach the edge of the lymph node you see them disappear inside. You follow, going deep into the center of the node. The macrophages are looking to find a special kind of cell, one that knows just what to do with the bit of vaccine material the macrophages want to show to them. From your previous journeys, you recognize this second variety of cell as a kind of lymphocyte. The two types of cells nuzzle right up against each other, touching close to the spot where the bit of germ material is on the macrophage surface. Clearly, the lymphocyte is interested in what the macrophage has to show it.

The lymphocyte is committing to memory the piece of vaccine material and will always remember and recognize it in the future. The macrophage accomplishes this trick by placing its catch in close proximity to special signal markers on its surface. When a lymphocyte sees those markers on the macrophage, it knows to pay attention to whatever particular thing lies next to them, because that special orientation indicates the thing is foreign, non-self.

The lymphocytes the macrophages are talking to are a special kind, called T-lymphocytes, or T-cells. They are central to immunity. Small and round in comparison to other cells, they are concentrated in lymph nodes. Some of them circulate in the blood, ranging throughout the body. You recall seeing a few of them sailing along with you in the bloodstream in chapter 1. In spite of their travels, they always eventually find their way back to a lymph node, using the extensive system of lymph canals as highways home.

As body cells go, some T-cells are very, very old. They can actually live for many years, perhaps even as long as we do. If you think for a moment about what immunity means, you can see why this is so. We need immunity to last as long as possible, and so-called memory cells are how this phenomenon happens. Besides being a Methuselah among cells, an individual memory T-cell is also relentlessly single-minded, being assigned only to remember a single foreign substance, to the exclusion of all else.

The immune response is varied and complicated, no doubt because the world of potential microscopic invaders is varied and complicated. We have to defend ourselves from bacteria like the H. flu germ. But we also must defend ourselves against a huge assortment of viruses, which are very different from bacteria, from tiny parasites, and even from the occasional fungus, like yeast. Even within the large category of bacteria, there is great diversity in the manner they use to attack the body, so our immune systems need to account for that. In spite of this diversity, the first step in the process for all of them is to enter the body and be tagged and cataloged as being from outside the body, as foreign. You have just seen how that happens.

For germs like H. flu, the principal arm of the immune system that deals with them is called the humoral system. It does its work by making what are called antibodies—protein substances that circulate in the blood and that serve as important weapons for attacking invaders. Inducing an antibody response in the child is the whole point of vaccination, because possessing that particular antibody protects the child from that particular infection. Doctors knew that and could even measure antibodies in a rough way, long before we knew how antibodies were even made. It is an example of a common phenomenon in medicine: often we can make practical use of a piece of knowledge even if we do not have the complete story explaining how it works.

Antibodies are made by another kind of cell, a lymphocyte cousin of the T-cell, called a B-cell. The B-cells are essentially factories for making antibodies. Our bodies have a huge assortment of B-cells, each of which has the ability to make a single kind of antibody, each slightly different from all the others, and there are millions of variations. Many B-cells live in the lymph nodes, but like the T-cells, they circulate in the blood from time to time. What the B-cell needs to know in order to do its job of making protective antibodies is this: Who is the enemy? It gets this information from its T-cell cousin.

Every B-cell has a single variety of antibody on its surface. To program the B-cell antibody factories, the controlling T-cells select, from the vast library of B-cells, one that has on its surface an antibody that is a good fit for the target. When it locates a perfect match, the T-cell tells this B-cell that this particular substance needs antibodies made against it, in this case, the bit of vaccine substance the nurse injected.

The newly selected B-cell then makes a trial run of antibody, a sort of rough draft effort. If that works, it then makes a final, refined version. A single cellular factory cannot make much antibody product. So, as part of this process, the B-cell also replicates, reproducing more cells just like itself, cells programmed to make the same antibody. After that happens, the B-cells are mature and ready to go if needed in the future. They become dormant factories, available whenever necessary to churn out massive amounts of the particular antibody for which they already have the blueprint. Like memory T-cells, B-cells are programmed only once against a single enemy.

The T-cells and B-cells look the same under the microscope. At the molecular level, though, they are quite different. Think of them as a family that has divided up the immunological work among themselves into a myriad of small teams. Scientists can tell which is which by looking for antibody on the surface for B-cells or for several other characteristic markers only T-cells have. T-cells themselves are divided into several different varieties, but for our purposes we do not need to concern ourselves with that further complexity.

The whole chain of events—macrophages arriving, scooping up the vaccine, and delivering it to the lymph node for processing—does take some time to happen. It is usually at least several weeks between vaccination and the first appearance in a child's circulation of antibodies against whatever was in the vaccine. You have now seen all you need to know about the initial stages of immunity, and you are ready to explore around the body to see if you can spot these immune cells at work.

A good place to do that is familiar territory—the middle ear. You can get there by finding your way to a small blood vessel and navigating to a handy exit point that will lead to his ear. You choose one of the largest of the boy's lymph nodes, a tonsil, both because that is near the middle ear and because it lets you appreciate once again the huge collection of lymphocytes, both T-cells and B-cells, standing guard against germ invasion. Children get a lot of sore throats, so the tonsils, like all the lymph nodes in that region, are prominent command centers for immunity. You squeeze out of one of the deep crypts in one of his tonsils and make your way back to the opening of his auditory tube. Things look completely normal there, and you duck inside.

Your journey up to the middle ear is uneventful. You soon find yourself back in its air-filled cavern. The arch above of interlinked bones is vibrating as it should, transmitting to the receiving hair cells on the other side of the oval window the vibrations that strike the boy's ear drum. This trip you are looking for other things, for ordinary phenomena that happen along the lining of the middle ear, things you missed before because there was so much drama absorbing your attention elsewhere.

As you skim slowly amid the cilia of the cavity wall, like an ocean fish passing through a kelp forest, you see a micro-drama taking place between an adventuresome bacterium that has successfully evaded the ear's defense system. A phagocyte is in hot pursuit of the germ, and you zoom down for a closer look. The bacterium is tumbling along the surface of the mucous layer, thus far managing to avoid being mired in it. This particular germ is large as bacteria go. It is lancet-shaped, being pointed on both ends and fatter in the middle. The phagocyte is determinedly crawling straight toward it and soon reaches it and tosses a membrane arm around both sides. It then extends these arms until the germ is surrounded, eaten. Even though this adventuresome germ made it into the middle ear, it will cause no trouble to the boy.

You next observe another micro-drama amid the cilia nearby. This one also stars bacteria and phagocytes, but this time the phagocytes appear less vigorous in their pursuit of the bacteria, which appear to be of a different species than the one you just saw meet his demise. These are small, pale, pear-shaped germs. Eventually a team of phagocytes surrounds and disposes of them, but it clearly was not as efficient a process as the first one. Why not?

You have just witnessed the benefits of having specific antibody. The first bacterium, the lancet-shaped one, was what is called a pneumococcus. It is a common inhabitant of the respiratory tract, especially the nasal cavity. As such, it is a very common cause of ear infections, because it is poised and ready to invade if the auditory tube malfunctions. It also has the disturbing tendency to invade a child's bloodstream and cause serious infection elsewhere in the body once it gains a foothold anywhere, such as in the ear. This is why we have a vaccine for it, and your friend's son had received it previously. It is not a perfect vaccine, since pneumococcus comes in many varieties and the vaccine only covers some of these, but it does help protect children against the most common ones.

Since he has been vaccinated against pneumococcus, his body has specific antibodies against it circulating in his blood. He also has a group of memory cells, primed and ready to pour out more antibody if the amount already present in his blood is not sufficient to get the job done. Some of these antibodies seep out of the wall of the middle ear. When a pneumococcus passes by, the antibody recognizes it and does its job.

Antibodies are proteins, tiny molecules. They are so tiny you cannot see them, even in your present microstate. You cannot see them, but medical researchers have the ability to see their structure. They are shaped like a Y, with two arms and a tail. Each of the arms has a zone that fits around the antibody's target like a lock and key. That target is determined back when the first responding cell processes it and presents it to a T-cell, along with the flag telling the T-cell to remember this thing as an enemy. An antibody molecule spends its entire career looking for just that one thing.

An individual antibody molecule lasts for a few weeks, then gets recycled by the body. The group of B-cell factories that made it will generally replace it with fresh antibody, since there is always a small number of them in production mode. Over time, these antibody factories do tend to fade away if there is no call from the body to produce their particular product. This is why many vaccines require a booster injection, often years later. The booster wakes up that particular set of B-cells, inducing them to make replacement cells to preserve the immune system's memory of that particular thing.

Once an antibody spies its target, it sticks to it extremely tightly with the two arms of its Y-shaped structure. After it does that, the tail part is sticking outward. At the molecular level, a germ coated with antibodies resembles a porcupine with the tails of antibodies protruding outward from its surface. Phagocytes have their own lock-and-key system, and the tail of an antibody is one of the strongest phagocyte attractants there is: as soon as a germ gets coated with antibodies, it is marked for destruction. This is how vaccination against pneumococcus, H. flu, or many other germs protects the child from disease. The infection never is allowed to take hold because the vigilant antibodies immediately see it and tag it.

The immune system has other ways of killing germs besides antibodies, which is why the other bacteria you saw, the ones to which the boy did not have specific antibodies, eventually got destroyed. It took them longer, but they got the job done. Those were just a few germs; when faced by a more massive invasion, a lack of antibodies against the invaders puts our bodies at a serious disadvantage.

Now that you have seen the practical importance of the immune system demonstrated in front of you, it is time to end your journey, exiting by your old, familiar route out the nose. But you have seen only a small part of this complex system at work, the part that relates to vaccination. To understand healing you should read about at least a few of the other components of this intricate chain of interconnected cellular and molecular events. It is well worth your time.

Up until now we have been talking mostly about antibodies, sub-stances manufactured and released by immune cells that target germs. That arm of the immune system is called the humoral arm. The word derives from centuries-old terminology relating to things secreted by the body, called body humors. There is another important component of hu-moral immunity, called the complement system.

Complement consists of a family of proteins that circulate in our blood. These proteins are activated during all inflammatory reactions in a chain reaction, cascading manner. Once activated, pieces of comple-ment proteins signal to the phagocytes what to attack by attaching to the invader, just as antibodies do. Complement is also one of the most potent chemical messages for calling new phagocytes to the scene. Antibody-coated germs are powerful complement activators, but many bacteria and viruses can start the cascade on their own.

Unlike the case with antibodies, complement does not need to have previously seen a germ to know it is a germ. This is because we humans carry in our genes a long, ancestral memory for germs, the result of eons of struggles with them. In some ways complement is not as potent as antibody is against particular germs, but it is useful and powerful stuff to have in our immune arsenal. Complement is what allowed the second germ-versus-phagocyte drama you just saw in the middle ear end in the destruction of the germ by the pursuing phagocytes.

Besides humoral immunity, there is also what we call called cell-me-diated immunity. It gets its name because it does not involve substances in the blood like antibodies or complement. The directors of cell-medi-ated immunity are members of the T-cell family. They play key roles in the immune drama, particularly against germs that have devised ways to escape antibody attack.

Many viruses succeed in getting inside our cells, where they can hide out from antibodies and phagocytes. It is an old tactic, sufficiently old that our bodies have devised a counterstrategy. The virus-infected cells can ex-press on their surface unique molecules that serve as distress signals, tell-ing the immune system they are infected, and thus giving away the hiding place of the viruses. Cells in the cell-mediated immune system, comprised of some kinds of lymphocytes and the aptly named natural killer cells, see the distress flare and respond. Unfortunately for the virus-infected cell, that response is to kill it, virus and all, but that sacrifice is for the good of the whole body.

Humoral versus cell-mediated immunity is one way to think about the immune response, but there is another useful way, too. We can divide the immune response into innate and acquired immunity. The antibody response is acquired immunity—a child is not born with it, but needs to develop it as her body encounters the wide variety of germs out there in the wide world. Childhood is preeminently the time for doing this, which is why children get sick a lot relative to adults. This is especially true for respiratory viruses; the average preschool child will get about one illness from these per month.

What we call innate immunity is what all of us are born with, the product of our shared genetic heritage of past battles with microbes. Complement is one component of innate immunity, as are some aspects of cell-mediated immunity, such as natural killer cells. Phagocytes are part of innate immunity, too: although acquired immunity makes their job easier, they still can function without it. As you saw, they were a bit slower at chasing down the other bacteria in the middle ear, but they still got them, because they were aided by complement.

A child's body has other components of innate immunity. Local immunity of the sort found on surfaces like the inside of the intestines, the middle ear, and the respiratory tract partly involves antibody, but there are other key aspects of immunity that we all have from birth. This is well demonstrated by what happens to people born with an inherited defect that prevents their cilia from working properly; they are often bothered by respiratory infections in the areas where cilia function is key, such as in the lungs and sinuses. It is fair to think of the skin as another component in local immunity, too, because it forms a tight barrier to keep bacteria out.

All these overlapping aspects of immunity working together keeping us healthy have served us well through the eons. It is the redundancy of the system that is most impressive—we have many ways of accomplishing the same thing. Our immune system is like an airplane with multiple, overlapping fallback systems: a problem in one aspect of our immune response can often be made up for by the actions of another one.

The immune system is truly a wonderful apparatus. Yet perhaps because of its multifaceted complexity, things can go wrong with immunity in spite of the redundant backup capacity. The system can become confused. Sometimes we want this, as when doctors manipulate immunity after transplanting an organ from one person into another person. This would not be possible if we were unable to tame immunity. There are other times, however, when a confused immune system causes major problems. The most important of these is when the system loses its ability to distinguish self from non-self, a condition called autoimmunity. In effect, the body attacks itself.

A good way to consider this issue is to ask why our immune system does not attack us all the time. One would think it should now and then. Most of the things that provoke an immune response are protein molecules, like the H. flu vaccine you saw injected into the boy's leg, and our bodies contain several hundred thousand different kinds of proteins. Yet our immune system does not seem to do this. Why not? The answer lies in understanding the phenomenon of tolerance; that is, how our immune systems tolerate and leave our own tissues alone. Scientists do not fully understand the phenomenon, but they know a great deal about how tolerance happens, even if they cannot explain why. They do know that, just as the body learns who the enemy is, it also learns, over time, who its friends are.

T-lymphocytes get their name from their original home in the body, an organ called the thymus, which is located in the center of the chest, just underneath the breastbone. This home base is where all T-cells are born and initially raised. Young, immature T-cells are as unruly and rambunctious as young children. They use their budding immunological skills to become sensitized, meaning poised to attack all manner of things, including those around them. Some of these immature T-cells become primed to attack the body's own cells.

Fortunately for us, these young rogue T-cells get weeded out of the pool of available T-cells long before they are able to leave the thymus gland and circulate the body, potentially causing harm. How this actually happens is unclear, but it is clear that the T-cells as a group learn to distinguish self from non-self through a random process of trial and error. It is intriguing that the developing T-cell system learns its job in a similar way to how young children learn—first trying something, having it corrected by those who know better, and then trying again.

The B-cells have their own rogue cells that need to be eliminated, too. The B-cells get their name for their original home base, the bone marrow, where they are born. As you read, our bodies have a huge population of them, each with a unique antibody coating on its surface. The arms of the Y structure of each antibody are slightly different; they are all like tiny keys searching for the proper lock, which they will attack by sticking to it. T-cells select from this army of eager B-cells the proper one with the best fit, the one that sticks the best.

Since the initial process of generating all these B-cells with their unique antibodies is random, it is only natural that some of these antibodies will fit best with some aspect of the body's own cells or with a protein that normally circulates in the blood. Were they to be released into the circulation, these errant B-cells would make antibodies that would attack ourselves, called autoantibodies. Fortunately, most of these potential autoimmune B-cells do not make it into the circulation. Again, it is not exactly clear how this happens, but immature B-cells that make autoantibodies self-destruct before they can cause harm.

In spite of these safeguards, a few of the T- and B-cells that are programmed to attack us do escape the lymphocyte nurseries. They can actually be detected in normal people. A principal reason they rarely cause further problems is that there is another layer of control; without T-cells orchestrating events and instructing them who to attack, they never cause trouble.

In your travels to the infected finger and to the burst appendix, you saw damaged tissues and the healing cleanup that followed. Sometimes such damaged bits of tissue have become altered by the inflammatory process in such a way that the macrophages, doing their janitorial task, may now see them as foreign. If that happens, the altered material might be processed just as the vaccine you saw was and then provoke an immune response. There is some evidence that this can happen; native body components get altered just enough to fool a macrophage into thinking they are foreign, and the resultant antibodies, now properly called autoantibodies, can then recognize and react against the original, normal component. As you will read later, this sometimes happens and can cause serious disease when it does.

Keeping our immune systems tolerant of our own tissues is a multilayered process, complete with several backup systems. But there are even more safeguards than these. Our bodies have still another strategy to keep the immune system from attacking its own cells—subterfuge. Although there are thousands upon thousands of proteins in our bodies, not all of them are "visible" to the T and B-cells. If a particular protein can remain hidden from them, they cannot mistakenly make antibodies against it. Our bodies use this tactic in several places, particularly in our nervous systems. By keeping the active cells of the immune system from finding these places, we can help prevent immunological mishaps.

Tolerance, in all its complicated glory, is so effective at preventing aberrant immune attack that some microorganisms, particularly parasites, have developed ways of taking advantage of it, tricking the immune system. These invaders appropriate some of the proteins found on the surface of normal body cells and stick them on their own surface, like camouflage. The immune cells often pass them by, thinking they are part of the home team and not one of the enemy.

These are just some examples of what we know of the phenomenon of tolerance, of the immune system learning not to burn down its own house. It has many other aspects that are still poorly understood and are far too complicated for our purposes here. What is useful to know is that this tolerance did not spring forth, fully formed, in our systems; rather, our bodies had to learn how to do it. This is important when we next consider autoimmunity, the problem of the body attacking itself. In those situations, the immune system either did not learn what it should have or forgot what it learned in the past.

There is a large number of what we call "autoimmune diseases." These mostly affect adults, but some can afflict children, too. Some cause problems in only one organ system, others cause widespread derangements in the body. As you would predict, the problems a particular autoimmune disorder causes depend very much on what particular body component is the target. If the target is only located in a single organ, the dysfunctional immune attack is confined to that organ; if the target is something widely distributed around the body, then there are problems everywhere.

One autoimmune disorder in particular is often seen in children—diabetes. The full name for it is diabetes mellitus, type 1. This distinguishes it from type 2 diabetes, a different disease that mostly occurs in adults. Diabetes is an example of a very restricted kind of autoimmunity, so restricted that there is no immune attack anywhere else in the body besides the pancreas. This tells us that the autoantibody in children with diabetes ought to be directed against something that is only in one place, and researchers have found this to be the case.

Most people know that diabetes is a problem involving the amount of sugar in the blood. Without treatment, there is too much sugar. Children with diabetes can go on to have other problems, but all of these stem from the abnormal blood sugar. The high sugar comes from a complete lack of the hormone insulin.

Insulin is made in the pancreas, the organ you passed by during your trip down your daughter's intestine. It is nestled inside a loop formed by the duodenum, the first part of the small intestine. Most of the pancreas is devoted to making enzymes, which it dumps into the intestine to help digest our food. Scattered throughout the pancreas, however, are tiny islands of cells—usually about a million or so—that have a very different job. They make several hormones and release them into the blood, one of which is insulin. Insulin does several things, but its best-known function is allowing body cells to transport sugar from the bloodstream inside the cells. Since glucose, a simple sugar, is a principal fuel our bodies burn for energy, insulin is a crucial hormone for life. In fact, we cannot live without it for very long.

Children who develop diabetes have antibodies that attack what are called the beta-cells, the cells in the pancreas that make insulin and live in those scattered islands in the pancreas. Slowly, typically over months at least and possibly longer, the beta-cells are all destroyed. At that point, the child can no longer make insulin and her blood sugar rises to danger-ous levels. Most of the time, it is only then that the child sees a doctor because this process causes no symptoms at all, so there is no reason to see the doctor. It is when the child finally has almost no circulating insulin that the symptoms begin: typically excessive thirst, frequent urination, excessive hunger, and weight loss. By the time parents bring their child to the doctor, there typically is little or no insulin left, and no way to get it back.

Just what the autoantibodies are attacking in the beta-cells is un-known. What is known is that we can detect in nearly all of these children autoantibodies that are directed against several things in the beta-cells, including insulin itself. The antibodies may be a result of the autoimmune process, not its cause, since, as you read previously, damaged tissues can result in autoantibodies, at least for a while. But whatever the original target is in the beta-cells, at present there is nothing we can do to stop it. Besides, by the time we know about it, the child's insulin is gone because the cells that make it have been destroyed.

What causes this to happen? After all, this is a very specific disorder. Why does a child's immune system become confused so as to attack this particular, very small part of the body? It appears that things in the environment may trigger the events, particularly certain kinds of common viral infections. We suspect this for several reasons. Diabetes has a seasonal variation that correlates with the occurrence of several common viruses, one of them an intestinal virus. Researchers are not sure what is happening, but they suspect that an initially normal antibody response to the infection becomes deranged and turns its attack on the beta-cells. This may be because there are some surface proteins on the virus that mimic those on the insulin-producing cells.

Of course this theory raises several obvious questions. If these sorts of viral infections are so common, why doesn't every child get diabetes? And why do not all those intricate control mechanisms you read of earlier snuff out the autoimmune process before it gets going? Why does the system fail here?

The answers to these questions most likely relate to inheritance, our genetic makeup. Even before doctors knew anything about beta-cell autoantibodies, we knew that diabetes, as well as all the other autoimmune disorders, tends to cluster in families. It is complicated, which is not surprising, considering how complicated the immune system is. Most relatives of a child with diabetes do not have diabetes, and many children who have diabetes have no one in the family with the problem. But when we look at a large population of people, diabetes and all the less common autoimmune disorders do tend to cluster in related people. Researchers have some idea which inherited traits are likely driving this association. As expected, the genetic differences are found among the genes that control our immune response.

All humans are related to each another, however distantly. We all share the same body parts, and if you look at these body parts under a microscope, they are put together the same way. If you take the comparison to an even smaller level, that of the individual molecules in and on the surface of our cells, you also find that many of them are absolutely identical. However, many of them are not identical.

Over the eons, molecules that do the same thing in the body have occasionally drifted away from each other in their fine structure—the genes that make them have mutated or changed just a bit. As long as the molecule does its job, these occasional variances are of no consequence; scientists can detect them with fancy tests, but we generally never know we have them. We find examples of this throughout our genetic makeup. Like all our other inherited genes, this process has affected the immune system.

As you read, tolerance of self is key to the proper functioning of our immune system, and the body has multiple ways of ensuring that this happens properly. One important aspect is how the immune cells, such as the macrophages and T-cells, do their job, which is to find, process, and present to the rest of the immune system things that are foreign and need to be attacked. The molecular toolkit in those who are more prone to develop autoimmune disease has a propensity to become confused, identifying self as non-self. The result is autoimmune disease.

Two things are important to remember in this picture. People with this higher risk of autoimmune problems like diabetes are not abnormal. They are entirely normal, just normal in a different way from other people. It is also clear that just having this propensity is not enough to guarantee a response—something else must trigger it, likely something from the outside, like an infection. The familial associations with autoimmunity are very like the associations we see with many other disorders, such as heart disease and cancer. All humans are related, and nearly alike, but we differ from each other biologically in some of the fine details.

Before we leave the immune system, we should consider another important example of how we came to understand it and manipulate it—organ transplantation. Early attempts at placing an organ from one person inside another all failed because the recipient rejected the donor organ. We made no progress until we understood the immune response, especially the phenomenon of tolerance.

Most of the proteins on the cellular surfaces in the body are identical or nearly so. But there is one important class of molecules that is typically dramatically different from person to person. These proteins are intimately connected with the immune system; they are called the MHC proteins, short for major histocompatibility complex. Identical twins have the same MHC markers. Because they are inherited, we share half of them with each of our parents, but because there are so many varieties of MHC proteins, unrelated people usually differ significantly from each other. The genetic mathematics of the situation dictate that nobody is a perfect match for anybody else.

Unless we intervene to stop it, the MHC protein differences cause transplant recipients to attack and destroy the transplanted organ. Over the years, transplant doctors have learned which MHC profiles are more accommodating to each other than others, and they strive to match the two. Not surprisingly, close relatives are nearly always better matches than total strangers, but even with a parent, child, or sibling as a donor, the match is not perfect—the recipient's immune system will still reject the new organ. It will, that is, unless we manipulate it.

Our tools to modify immunity are blunt ones. We would like to have ways of convincing the body that the new organ is part of the same team, confusing the recipient's immune system enough to accept it and include it under the same tolerance umbrella granted to the other organs. Someday we may accomplish that, but we have a long way to go before we get there. For now, we have drugs that suppress immunity in various ways. We often cannot completely prevent rejection, but the goal is to keep it under control so that it does not harm the transplanted organ or the rest of the recipient's body.

Some of these drugs suppress all immunity, shutting down everything. For many years after transplantation began, that was all we had. Now we have other drugs that are more specific, especially ones that target how the various subclasses of T-cells work. As you would imagine, the problem with all these drugs is that we need our immune system in order to survive. The bacteria you saw in your daughter's large intestine would quickly invade if she had no immunity at all, as would all manner of germs that live in the environment. We know from practical experience that even our most powerful antibiotics often do not clear a patient's infection if there is a serious problem with that person's immune system. Transplant doctors are forever juggling the doses of the medicines, striving to find the lowest possible doses that will keep rejection at bay but still allow enough immune function to keep the person safe from infection. It is a very difficult tightrope to walk.

The immune system is central to how your child heals. In the best of scenarios, it makes it so your child hardly needs to heal at all, because her immunity prevents infection in the first place. Our experience with many vaccines has shown this is possible; many infections that once killed children by the thousands—like diphtheria, tetanus, and whooping cough—or injured them for life—like polio—are rarities today. If your child does get an infection, a well-functioning immune system is essential for controlling it. A good way to think of antibiotics is not that they cure infection but rather that they assist the immune system in doing so. The two work together.

Since immunity is so important to your child's health, is there anything you can do to strengthen it and make it work better? It would certainly help healing if you could. A myriad of late-night television infomercials and Internet Web sites promise products that do just that. In fact, "strengthening the immune system" seems to be a near-universal claim of dietary supplements and herbal remedies. It would be a wonderful thing if these claims were correct—so, are they?

Answering this question would be another book, but the short answer is that there are no convincing data that anything can help the immune system in that way. It is not something medical researchers have ignored; they have been working on the possibility for many years, particularly in regard to cancer research (more on that in a later chapter). The bottom line is that the best ways to keep your child's immune system working well are the commonsense ones: good diet, exercise, and sufficient sleep, since there is evidence that deficiencies in these can cause problems. Of course, every parent already knows that.

· 6 ·

When the Environment Attacks:
Allergies and Other Encounters

 $\mathcal{S}$ everal of the previous chapters have shown you what a child's body does when germs attack, how she fights them off and how she heals afterward. Not all outside threats to a child's body come from germs—there are plenty of other things in the world around her that can cause trouble. Some of these behave the same for all children; others are issues only for children particularly susceptible to their effects.

Imagine it is August. Your son from the first chapter, the aspiring carpenter, has the sniffles. He appears fine otherwise; he has no cough, no sore throat, and no fever. He is not complaining about anything hurting. His appetite and energy are the same. The only things you notice besides his runny nose are that his eyes are a little red and there is a suggestion of a darker blush of color under both of them, something you did not notice until his visiting grandmother pointed it out to you.

Whatever is going on, it is clear that his nose is central to the process. Since that is territory you now know well, we should return there to see what is causing his symptoms. You enter one of his nostrils just as before and travel down to where the mucous layer drapes itself across the cells and is pushed along by all those beating strands of cilia waving in unison.

You recall that the surface last time was pale pink in color. The mucus that coated it was thin and nearly translucent. In contrast, when your two-year-old had the viral infection, the cold that ultimately led to his ear infection, the mucus was thick, gooey, and yellowish-green. There also was a huge amount of it. What you see now is a combination of both those situations; the stuff is watery thin and looks clear, but there is a massive amount of it. When you saw it in his normal nose it was a stately, slow-moving stream. Now, on your microscopic level, it is a flood, a rushing river swirling around the base of his nasal hairs.

Any disaster movie's stock footage of a flood shows images of houses, cars, and trees being washed away. Hovering above this torrent, you see a similar thing, only in this case, clumps of cells torn from the bottom stand in for the buildings in the movie. In spite of the fury of the mucous waters you notice it is not murky—you can see clear through to the bottom—but the bottom does not look like the surface you remember from your earlier trip, when his nose was normal.

The normal pinkish surface is now bright red. It is also swollen and boggy looking, with its surface rising to a height many times what it was before. Whatever is causing all this mischief in your son's nose, it is obvious that the answers lie down there, below the surface of his nasal mucosa. If you want to understand it, you will need to dive down and have a look around. The safest place to do that appears to be an eddy in the river on the lee side of a nose hair, so down you go.

When you plunge through the waves, you are momentarily swept along with all the other debris, but your engines are powerful enough to escape the pull of the current, and you drive your craft quickly to the bottom. There the current is gentler, and you are able to bump along among the cilia. You immediately see they have been severely affected by the torrent, and many are broken off. Worse, there are large patches on the bottom where there is no cilia layer at all, because the cells that sprout the cilia, the epithelial cells, have been ripped up and swept downstream. You will need to go deeper still to investigate, so you select a spot between two surviving epithelial cells and squeeze your vessel between them. You are no longer a submarine, and now you use your all-terrain vehicle mode to crawl between and over the cells.

You have many questions to answer. The first of these is from where all the mucus is coming. Is it coming from somewhere back up in the nose, beyond where you could see, as when a thunderstorm high in the mountains causes a flash flood in a canyon below? It certainly appeared that could be the case when you were flying above it. Now, however, you see this is not so. The river is not flowing down from the dark recesses of your son's upper nasal passages. It is coming from all around you, welling up like a spring-fed river.

Scattered around you are some oblong structures, crypts in the surface layer of the lining of his nose, which extend downward into the underlying tissue. They are perhaps ten or twenty cells deep and narrower at the point where they open outward to the surface. They resemble bags with their drawstrings partly cinched closed at the exit point. These bags are full to overflowing with mucus, which is pouring out of their openings, feeding the rushing stream above you. You approach one of these structures, careful not to actually get inside one, because you would certainly be washed back out into the flood if you did so. You see the cells lining these bags are not like those on the surface above you. These cells have no cilia and are shaped a little differently from ciliated cells.

You are looking at a mucous factory. The job of the cells working in this factory is to make mucus and release it into the sack, after which it gets pushed out to the surface. The factory clearly seems to be making too much product, but really these cells are just doing their job, although they are doing it far more excessively than they should.

You next turn your attention to some of the other cells around you and see some familiar sights, a reminder that a child's tissues respond to a wide variety of challenges in very similar ways. The repertoire of these cellular actors—like all actors—is limited to what they know how to do.

Recall what you saw in your son's inflamed finger. Then his problem was that germs carried beneath the protective layer of his skin by a tiny wood splinter initiated the process of inflammation, the cascade first of local events that soon ballooned to involve cellular actors recruited to the drama from distant parts of the body. In this case there is no splinter and no germs, either, although you can see how easily germs might penetrate down here, since the protective layer of ciliated cells is gone in so many places. Of course to do so they would first have to brave the mucous flood and avoid being washed away.

You are in sodden, swollen tissues. Sometimes swelling comes from the enlargement of the cells that live in the involved tissues, but most times swelling is caused by leakage of fluid from surrounding capillary blood vessels into the tissue, pushing the cells there farther apart. That was the case in the inflamed finger, and that is what you see now. You see that the meshwork of capillaries is riddled with huge holes, like cheesecloth. Fluid from the blood is streaming out, and some of the holes are so large that an occasional red blood cell drifts through them. These are familiar sights.

Inflamed tissues get their red color from red blood cells. The process of inflammation draws more blood to the site by increasing the diameter of the blood vessels. That is one cause of the redness. But redness also comes from blood cells that have leaked out of capillaries. That is why, even after the fires of inflammation have cooled, there is often some residual discoloration at the site that takes a while to disappear—those errant red blood cells need to be broken down and hauled away by the cellular cleanup crew.

As you look around at this particular example of inflamed tissue, you notice that it seems more boggy with fluid even than the finger did at its worst. On the other hand, there are clear differences in the kinds of cells roaming around from those you saw in the infected finger. For one thing, you do not see many phagocytes, which you saw in abundance in the finger. There are some here and there but not many. This makes sense because an important job of the phagocytes is hunting down and killing germs, aided by the immune and complement systems, posting all those red flags on the germs, marking them for attack and destruction. Since you see no germs anywhere, it is logical that there are few phagocytes about.

You do observe two varieties of cells you have not seen before. They look a lot like the phagocytes from your past explorations, but they are not quite the same. Are they related, perhaps? Both are more or less the same size as the phagocytes. You can see right through them, since they are translucent, but when you look closely, you see that both types have several hundred granules that look like pebbles scattered throughout their insides. Although they look similar in most ways, you can see they behave a little differently.

One variety has new representatives arriving constantly via the nearby capillaries; they stop, grab onto the capillary wall, and then crawl out to join the drama just as you saw phagocytes do. The other variety appears to be a normal resident here, because you see no fresh examples appearing. Both of them are busy dumping the contents of their packets of granules into the area around them, and the whole area is littered with cells that have already spent their granular ammunition and are merely lying about, waiting to be dismantled and carted away. Both cell types are principal players in the cellular drama we call allergy, and your son's nose is the stage for that very common play. At least 10 percent of people have nasal allergies, although the severity varies widely from person to person.

The resident cell, the one not getting continual reinforcements, is called a mast cell. Mast cells are central to how the phenomenon of allergy works. They are born in the bone marrow, which is where blood cells like phagocytes come from. But although they are related to blood cells, they are only cousins. They are not fully mature when they leave their birthplace; that happens later when they find their particular duty station in the body. The places naturally rich in mast cells tend to be areas where the outside world impinges closely on the body's interior world. These places include the skin and the lining of the upper airway, such as the nose.

A good way to think of a mast cell is that of an alert guard, armed with a host of biological weapons, who doggedly waits for a very specific target. When it feels that particular enemy touch the tripwires on its surface— something we call activation—it launches the arsenal—the whole load. These substances cause all the symptoms we experience as allergies.

Foremost among the things an activated mast cell lets loose into its surrounding tissue is a molecule called histamine. Mast cells tend to congregate around small blood vessels. When they release histamine, it causes a large increase in the diameter of nearby blood vessels, resulting in engorgement of the vessels with blood. Histamine also creates those holes you are seeing in the capillaries by opening up gaps between the cells lining the vessel. Together, this causes immediate swelling and, usually, redness. In the skin, mast cells also gather near nerve endings, where released histamine causes the nerve sensation we know as itching.

Histamine is an incredibly powerful substance. If large amounts of it get into the bloodstream it can cause a catastrophe. The sudden increase in blood vessel diameter does the same thing to a person's blood pressure that quadrupling the diameter of cold water pipes would do to your household water pressure: a fixed amount of fluid now needs to occupy a significantly larger space, so there is less fluid to go around. As a result, pressure falls dramatically, and a sudden, huge fall in blood pressure has profound effects on the body, some of them serious.

Histamine can have serious effects on breathing, too. It can bring on swelling of the tongue and soft tissues around the back of the throat, blocking airflow. It causes intense tightening of those tiny muscular nooses you saw around the bronchioles in chapter 3, causing an asthma attack. It is this property of histamine that forms the link between some people with allergies and asthma.

Mast cells release many other substances besides histamine when they are activated. These include enzymes, cousins of the digestive enzymes you saw in the stomach and small intestine. Except in this case, the enzymes actually go to work digesting some of the cellular tissues in the area, leading to damage. The action of these enzymes also triggers the same cascade of events you witnessed in the infected finger, which called other actors in the inflammation drama to the scene.

These are the immediate things mast cells do, things that occur within an hour or so. But there is more: mast cells also initiate an entirely different set of events, actions that fan the flames of inflammation even higher. After they have released their prepackaged granules full of histamine, they switch on dormant molecular machinery, which manufactures even more substances, which draw still more cells there. Some of these later arrivals are the familiar phagocytes; others are those cells you saw crawling out of the capillary blood vessels. In such a scenario, an initial set of annoying symptoms can easily become a chronic situation that feeds on itself.

What your son is experiencing are the messy results of mast cell activation—runny nose, itchy eyes, and tissues in his nose so swollen that he cannot breathe through it. How and why do mast cells do this to some, but not all of us, and, most importantly, what can we do about it?

The mast cell is really part of the immune system. In the last chapter you read about antibodies, those substances in the blood that attach themselves to foreign invaders. They are highly specific and only attack one thing. Mast cells are completely covered with a very special sort of antibody called immunoglobulin E. This antibody mostly targets environmental irritants like ragweed pollen, house dust, or animal dander. People who have allergies have their mast cells coated with this kind of antibody. It is highly specific; just like their cousins, the B-cells, each mast cell has only one target, and people who are allergic to one thing are not necessarily allergic to anything else, although they tend to be.

Think of a mast cell as resembling a picture of one of those World War II–era sea mines, a ball of explosives with spines sticking out all over it. The spines are the immunoglobulin E molecules. When the target against which the mast cells are primed touches the surface, the mine explodes and dumps out its granular contents.

The tendency to have allergies runs in families. This is not surprising. Allergies are closely tied to the immune system, and, as you read in the last chapter, the details of how the immune system operates vary from person to person. Some people quite happily live surrounded by ragweed plants; others begin to sneeze and to have a runny nose if they only drive on a country road in August with the car window down for a minute. The latter people have mast cells in their noses charged and ready to explode, the former do not.

How can we treat allergic symptoms? What can we do to make your son feel better? From what you have seen, you might imagine several ways we might help. The simplest way of reducing allergic symptoms is to avoid whatever your child is allergic to. That is easy if it is cats, less so if it is airborne pollen that is everywhere during certain seasons. Still, avoidance is best if possible. At any rate, having seen enough, you head for home.

For many years we have been able to treat allergies by blocking the action of a main culprit in the symptoms, histamine, which is why the drugs are called antihistamines. There are many on the market, but the most widely used for decades has been a drug called diphenhydramine, brand name Benadryl. It is a very potent histamine blocker. As you read, however, mast cells release many other things besides histamine, and antihistamines do nothing to stop the effects of those other substances. In addition, many of the older antihistamines can have unpleasant side effects, the most common of which is drowsiness. We now have a newer generation of antihistamines that are much less likely to do this, such as loratadine (a common brand is Claritin) and cetirizine (Zyrtec being a common brand), but blocking histamine effects is not the entire answer for many children.

We have additional allergy treatments that block the actions of the other actors in the play. One of these, cromolyn (brand name Nasalcrom), interferes with the ability of mast cells to release their granules. Another, montelukast (brand name Singulair) blocks a member of the second wave of substances the mast cells manufacture once their histamine is gone. Finally, we can use one of the many members of the steroid class of medicines, typically as a nasal spray. Steroids nonspecifically dampen all aspects of the immune reaction, allergies included. Common brand names of these medications are Flonase, Nasacort, Nasonex, and Rhinocort. These medicines usually help the symptoms, but sometimes that kind of global inhibition of local immunity produced by steroids is not the best answer.

For some children, we have a final mode of therapy that can be quite effective, although time consuming and mildly uncomfortable for the child. It is called desensitization therapy, and the goal is to confuse the child's mast cells. The principle is that repeated exposure to the offending agent by injection, in initially small but steadily increasing doses, keeps the child's mast cells from behaving in such an explosive manner. In effect, they become more tolerant of it. Desensitization does not work for every allergic substance or for every child, and the course of shots usually must be given weekly for several months before the child gets any benefit. The shots then typically must be continued for at least several years afterward. Most doctors reserve this kind of therapy for children who have more severe allergies, ones that affect more than their noses.

For your son to heal completely from the problems you saw in his nose, the allergic cycle of primed mast cells reacting to whatever he is allergic to must be broken. This can happen by removing the trigger—such as when all the ragweed plants freeze in winter or when you give away your cat to a relative—or by one or more of the several treatments I described earlier. Once the pattern of continual, self-reinforcing irritation and inflammation stops, the tissues in his nose quickly heal. The blood vessels stop leaking, mucous production slows back to normal, and the roving inflammatory cells wander off somewhere else, now that there is nothing summoning them there.

In the finger, the result of the battle between germs and the inflammatory system inevitably left a few gaps and holes in the tissues that needed to be repaired by filling them in with fibroblasts. If the holes are big enough, the fibroblasts make a scar. Unless the allergic process is very severe, this does not happen for allergies. If you can control those pesky mast cells, his nose will heal back to just the way it was before his runny nose began.

Many people have no allergies at all to the common things around us. But even for those fortunate souls, there are things in the environment that usually provoke a similar response. You might thing of them as substances to which nearly all of us are all allergic, because they provoke an allergy-like reaction in most people who are exposed to them. Such a substance is the oil found in the poison ivy plant.

Not everybody reacts to poison ivy, and their sensitivity varies, but most of us do break out in a rash if enough of the oil from the plants gets on our skin. When it does, it causes a red, itchy, and often blistering rash. If you were to travel beneath the skin of someone with poison ivy, the rash would look very familiar to you. There are the same leaking capillaries engorged with blood and the same inflammatory cells recruited by the substances the mast cells release. Since there are no mucous-secreting cells in the skin, that part is different from what you saw in the nose, but the rest would look very much the same.

The skin is rich in mast cells, too, which is why patients with allergies can get rashes. As with plant pollens, children vary in their propensity to this. But the oil in poison ivy (called urushiol) is so good at sensitizing mast cells that few of us can avoid having it happen to us. It is something to which the majority of us become allergic if we are exposed. Our first exposure primes the mast cells, later ones produce the rash.

Allergies are uncomfortable and annoying. For some people they are so severe they can even be life threatening. Why do many of us have them? Do they serve any useful purpose at all? We do not know the answer to those questions. Certainly the response of the lungs to a hefty dose of histamine—an asthma attack—does not seem particularly helpful to the body, and it can be dangerous. Yet there is evidence, still very incomplete, that some of the substances released by mast cells aid cellular healing, particularly in helping to grow new blood vessels. These materials also may have some benefit in fighting off parasites, such as intestinal worms. These days, few of us in Western societies are troubled by worms, but many thousands of years ago this was not the case. So these annoying reactions may have been of real benefit to our ancestors.

Allergy is just one of the innumerable ways the environment can cause unwanted effects on a child's body. The phenomenon of allergy reminds us that although doctors can make useful generalizations about how things usually will turn out based upon what we know, it is the unique properties of each child's body that ultimately determine the outcome. Each child is an individual.

Another important way our bodies encounter the environment is through what we eat. As you saw, the digestive system contains many feet of intestine. This means there is a sustained opportunity for whatever we swallow to interact with our insides as it passes through. Any parent with more than one child knows that this process affects each child differently. Usually these differences do not matter much, but sometimes they do. Our next scenario will show you what can happen on one of these occasions.

Imagine your sister is visiting you for a month and has brought her two children along to play with their cousins. You have not seen her or her children for more than a year. The two of you are sitting in the kitchen looking at old photographs and watching your son and his cousin play outside.

Both are boys of the same age. In the past they were nearly the same size, both in height and weight, but now you can clearly see that your son is several inches taller than his cousin. Even more obvious is the difference in build. Your son has broader shoulders and a fuller chest; in contrast, the other boy has thin, bony shoulders and spindly arms and legs. You assume this is just an innate difference in body type beginning to show itself as they grow. Then you glance down at the photographs taken during past, shared vacations; a year ago the two might have been taken for twins, and the year before that, too.

Your sister has followed your thoughts, as sisters will. She points out the obvious contrast between the two boys now. In fact, she has been worried about it for some time. Her son generally seems well and continues to have what looks like a normal appetite to her. However, he has begun to complain now and then about vague pains in his belly. He also has had several bouts of diarrhea during the past several months. These resolved on their own and both your sister and the child's doctor attributed the symptoms to stomach flu. Now she is not so sure about that.

After talking about it for a while, she decides she does not want to wait a month to take him back to his regular doctor, and she asks you to make an appointment with your children's physician while they are still visiting. Later in the week the two of you and her son visit your doctor. Before the appointment, your sister collects some actual weight measurements of her son for the past several years.

The doctor listens to your sister's story and examines her child. What impresses the doctor most is a chart she makes of the child's growth. Children do come in many sizes and grow at different rates, but years of measuring children have given doctors an excellent understanding of what is normal. The most important thing to look at when you make a growth chart is not the absolute number in terms of height or weight, but how it has changed over time. A progressive slippage of growth rate causes concern, and that is what has happened to your nephew, especially during the past two years.

The doctor orders some tests. Her main concern is that your nephew's digestive system is not using the food that he eats correctly, something called malabsorption. She is also concerned that his chronic, intermittent diarrhea and belly pain may be a sign of problems in his digestive tract, since children with malabsorption often have those symptoms.

Before those tests come back, though, you decide what would really help both of you understand what is going on is a trip to your nephew's digestive tract. After all, you have been there before, when your daughter had appendicitis, so you know the terrain. Since your exploration vehicle has room for two, you invite your sister to come along.

The first part of your road trip takes you through his mouth to the back of his tongue. Then it is over his epiglottis, closed now because it is protecting his airway from errant bits of food and other swallowed things. Poised at the back of his throat, you wait for the next time he swallows. When he does, you ride the wave of muscular contraction in his esophagus down toward his stomach. When you reach the end of his esophagus you pop through the opening in the ceiling of his stomach, glide through the air for a second, and then plop down in a puddle of stomach juice.

This is all new to your sister, but to you everything in the stomach looks completely normal: the walls of the stomach have a nice, healthy pink color, and they glisten in your light, wet with digestive juices. You dive down and head for the pylorus, the stomach outlet valve. After a several minute wait, it opens and you pass through, along with a portion of the stomach contents.

You are once again in the first portion of the small intestine, the place where the digestive enzymes from the boy's pancreas and bile from his liver squirt into the stream from the opening overhead. The river of food itself is too thick and murky to let you see much of the intestinal wall, so you navigate to a quiet eddy next to the wall to get a closer look. Here things look decidedly different from the situation when you visited your daughter's digestive system before she got appendicitis.

The wall of the normal intestine then showed a soft, undulating surface of successive folds. Your closer inspection revealed that, although the surface looked smooth at a distance, close to the actual lining of the small intestine, it was definitely not smooth; rather, it consisted of a dense array of fingerlike projections. These are called villi, and they resemble tufts of hair. Each of them was coated with many hundreds of individual intestinal cells.

The outer layer of cells covering the villi, the ones directly facing the food stream in the intestine, are where the actual absorption of nutrients into the system happens. It makes sense why nature would put the absorbing machinery on all those villi, because it allows the wall of the intestine to have a much larger surface area than if the walls were smooth. More surface area means more lining cells, which in turn leads to more absorption of food. The absorbing cells themselves also use a trick to increase their own surface area: they extend masses of tiny projections, called microvilli, because they are smaller versions of the villi that line the walls. The overall effect is like the surface of a brush, which is why this region is commonly called the "brush border."

There are other cells within the villi. There are specialized cells for transporting the various kinds of nutrients where they need to go. Also, the food stream in the intestine is loaded with bacteria, so the entire region needs to have frequent outposts of the immune system to deal with the occasional germ that makes it through the brush border and gets inside. Like the places in the ear and the respiratory tract you have visited, the intestines need active and strong local immunity as a barrier to germ invasion.

You remember all these things from your visit to your daughter's normal intestine. What you are seeing now, however, is very different. When you approach the wall, the first thing you notice is that nearly all the tufts of villi hair are gone. Instead of an extensive range of steep, tightly pack hills coated with intestinal cells, you see a flat prairie. It does have a meager coating of food-absorbing cells, but there are also places when there are very few or even none of these. You zoom closer for a better look.

Up close, you see the villi have been chopped off, as if someone took a lawnmower and shaved them off to make everything smoother. When you shine your light down into the crypts, the clefts at the bases of and between the villi, you are surprised to see plenty of absorbing cells. These crypts are the nurseries for absorbing cells, which normally last several days. It looks like the nurseries are in overdrive, desperately trying to make new cells to replace the losses. Just from what you have seen thus far it makes sense that the boy has not been growing—a large number of the cells he needs to absorb his food are simply gone. The fact that his body is obviously creating as many new ones as possible suggests that they must be getting destroyed by something as part of an ongoing process.

You dive down and land on one of the chopped-off villi, since that seems to be where the problem lies. Passing between two of the feeble remnants of the absorbing cell system, you make your way deeper into the wall of the boy's small intestine. When you get there, you see some familiar friends.

What you see are the usual players in immunity and inflammation. There are many T-cells, macrophages, phagocytes, and even the occasional mast cell. Clearly, all these cells are there, doing what they think is their job, but why have they come? There are no germs around, so infection is not the answer. The scene, although familiar to you in some ways, also is different. It looks much older than any cellular battlefield you have seen before. It does not have the red-hot look of the fierce immune and inflammatory fights you saw before in both the ear and the finger. Here things resemble old battlefield photographs of World War I, with the terrain scarred from many earlier battles, and the cells you see around you go about their tasks more listlessly. What you are looking at is the result of many months of chronic inflammation.

As you and your sister survey the torn-up landscape, it is clear to you what is happening here. It is also obvious it has been going on for some time. Something is destroying the absorbing cells and the villi on which they normally live, and that destruction is interfering with your nephew's normal digestion. No wonder he has belly pain now and then. Looking around you at all the mess, it is amazing he does not have pain all the time. If he cannot absorb his food, he cannot grow normally.

He also has had periodic troubles with diarrhea for many months. There are many possible causes for diarrhea, but a common one is when unabsorbed nutrients make it all the way through the digestive tract to the colon, the large intestine. When that happens, the mixture is too rich for the large intestine's normal functions, and the result is loose, watery stools—diarrhea—often accompanied by belly cramps. Since the absorptive capacity of the cells in the small intestine is diminished, this is what is happening to the boy.

You can see what is happening; what you don't know is why this is happening. Are the absorbing cells being directly attacked and killed by something, and are all the immune and inflammatory cells there to try to fight off whatever that is? Or are the absorbing cells simply innocent bystanders, injured and killed by what a general might call friendly fire? There are examples of both possibilities in the annals of human disease, and either could result in your nephew's symptoms.

A pathologist, an expert in how disease affects tissues, can look through a microscope at what you are seeing and identify the problem. In fact, that is how we diagnose your nephew's condition: we pass a thin tube all the way down into the small intestine, take a small sample of the intestinal wall, called a biopsy, and send it to a pathologist. (The procedure is painless, but children are given sedatives to keep them comfortable.) The flattened villi, increased absorbing-cell production by the crypts, and chronic inflammation just below the surface are characteristic of a disorder called celiac disease, or sprue. It is also called gluten-sensitive enteropathy, a name that accurately describes what causes it. "Enteropathy" is just a fancy way of saying something is wrong with the intestines. What is important is that exposure to gluten causes it.

Gluten is a protein component of wheat, and there is also some in barley and rye. When people with celiac disease eat something with gluten in it, their small intestines react in the way your nephew's did. It is relatively common, affecting perhaps 1 percent of the population. However, the severity of an individual's symptoms is extremely variable. Some people have no symptoms at all; others have much more severe symptoms than your nephew does. Researchers do not understand the reason for this wide variability, although clearly some people are more sensitive to gluten than are others.

Even though we know that gluten triggers the symptoms, exactly how it does this is less clear. It appears the gluten provokes an immune response similar to the ones you have seen earlier. Once that initial event happens, intestinal cells are damaged, and autoantibodies are formed that mistakenly target some of the components on the intestinal cells. We can measure these aberrant antibodies with a blood test; if they are present, that fact plus the biopsy result confirms the diagnosis.

The cellular details of celiac disease are still foggy. What is clear is that the process is closely linked to the immune system. That means it is connected to heredity, because the fine details of how our immune systems work are also tied to our heredity. It is an autoimmune disease. As you read in chapter 5, autoimmune diseases are those in which the body mistakenly attacks and damages its own tissues. In this case, the target is the absorbing cells themselves. You should not be surprised that people with celiac disease and their families have a higher incidence of other autoimmune disorders.

Celiac disease is unique in that it is the rare autoimmune disease for which we know the specific trigger—gluten. The relationship between an environmental exposure and the misguided immune response is clear in this case. It is likely that most if not all other autoimmune problems, like type 1 diabetes in the previous chapter, have some kind of environmental trigger, too; we just do not know what they are yet. Even if we find the triggers, it may well be that the autoimmune response continues by itself even when the trigger is removed. Fortunately, this is not the case with celiac disease—we have an effective treatment for it.

The treatment for celiac disease is eliminating gluten from the diet. Once the trigger is gone, the intestine nearly always heals completely, especially in a child like your nephew. An adult who has had the problem for many years and has unknowingly continued to eat gluten may not be able to heal completely, but removing gluten from the diet always improves the situation dramatically. A gluten-free diet is not simple to follow, but millions of people do it successfully. The key is not only eliminating obvious sources of wheat, rye, and barley, but also knowing the foods in which these grain products may be hiding, such as many processed foods.

This chapter illustrated several ways in which the environment, the world around us, can attack a child's body. Sometimes such attacks are straightforward—everything from sunburn to bug bites to lightning strikes is easy to understand. But other times the environment is only the initiator of problems, and it is the body itself that continues them.

· 7 ·

Fevers, Aches, and Itches: Where Do Symptoms Come From?

𝒮n all our scenarios, you encountered symptoms, like your son's painful finger or your daughter's nausea. Your explorations showed you the places in their bodies where the causes of those symptoms must lie. Yet you saw nothing that explained where they came from, or why they disappeared when the child's problem improved. Surely the symptoms going away was part of the healing process, evidence that things were going well, but how did that happen?

This chapter is about the common subjective feelings children have when they are ill—what causes them, how those feelings go away, and why, sometimes, they can linger long after all other aspects of the problem have healed. Because symptoms are subjective and thus cannot be seen directly, there is no exploration you can undertake that will demonstrate them to you. So for this chapter, your vehicle must remain in the garage.

By long tradition doctors have used the word symptom a little differently than nonphysicians do. By strict definition, a symptom is something felt or perceived by the patient; it cannot be observed or measured by anyone else. By these criteria, pain and nausea are symptoms, but fever is not, because a high temperature can be demonstrated to be there (or not) with a thermometer. The same is true for cough, vomiting, diarrhea, and swelling; because another person can observe these things, the strictly correct medical term for them is not symptoms but rather signs. To nonphysicians this distinction can seem like splitting hairs. For our purposes, we will lump these two categories together, as most people do.

PAIN

Pain, in all its varieties and subtleties, is among the most complex of human symptoms. It has been described in uncounted ways by writers and portrayed by actors, but we read or view these characterizations through the lens of the pain we ourselves have experienced. Even though we all have felt pain, and in that sense, have shared the experience with all other humans, it is also unique to us. Pain is both universal and profoundly personal.

Pain is not limited to humans, of course. All mammals certainly feel pain. Some aspects of the pain response reach far down below mammals in the animal kingdom to quite primitive creatures. How these creatures perceive it, if that is even the right word, is mysterious, but this observation tells us pain has been with us for many eons. That fact alone should tell us it must serve some important purpose.

All of us know that pain comes in many forms. There is the sharp pain from stepping on a tack. There is the vague, dull aching of a twisted knee, the cramping pain in the lower abdomen that comes with the flu, the pounding inside the skull of a migraine headache, the gnawing pain of a toothache. There is the restless pain that persists in spite of what positions you take, as well as the pain that only relents when you lie completely still. All of us could think of many more examples.

Because pain is so complicated, doctors are trained to sort it out using a series of simple questions we ask patients about their experience. These defining terms include the following:

1. Location: Where does it hurt?
2. Radiation: Does the pain go anywhere, or does it stay in one spot?
3. Quality: Describe the pain in your own words.
4. Quantity: Rate the pain on a ten-point scale, with zero being no pain and ten being the worst pain you have ever felt.
5. Duration: How long have you had it? Is it always present, or does it come and go?
6. Frequency: If it comes and goes, how often does it do that and how long does it last when it is present?

7. Aggravating factors: Does anything make it worse?
8. Alleviating factors: Does anything make it better?
9. Associations: Does the pain seem related to other symptoms in any way?

This all sounds very logical, and your answers to these questions are very helpful to the doctor in figuring out what is causing your pain. Certainly the location of your daughter's pain helped the doctor decide she had appendicitis. Young children, of course, can tell the doctor little about it other than its location, and infants cannot help at all, other than crying to let us know they hurt somewhere.

Before your explorations of the body's microscopic world, you might have found these general comments sufficient. Now, though, I expect you want to know more precisely just where the different sorts of pain come from—just how, for instance, your son's swollen finger made him experience pain. You also want to know how pain relates to healing. Does it help your child heal, or might he heal better without it?

The simplest pain to consider is superficial pain, such as a prick from a rose thorn. On your visit to your son's finger you actually passed some of his pain-reporting systems. I did not point out to you at the time the dense network of nerve fibers, but they were all around you, just under his skin. Think of this network as an intricate grid of electrical wires, because that is what nerve signals are made of—electricity.

These wires are of several kinds, but there are two principal ones. They differ in how well insulated they are. Instead of the plastic insulation that protects electrical wires, the body uses a substance called myelin to insulate the neural wiring. Some wires are more tightly wrapped with myelin than others. Some nerve fibers have no myelin at all. The more wrapping, the faster the electrical signal travels, so myelinated fibers transmit signals faster than those without myelin.

The nervous system uses a series of switching stations to pass a signal from, for example, the end of your finger to your brain. The first of these are in the spinal cord. When you prick your finger, an electrical signal goes from a nerve fiber there, up your arm, and on to a relay station in the spinal cord in your neck. From there, it continues on up your spinal cord to your brain. What happens to it when it reaches your brain is fascinating—and complicated.

Pain is a subjective feeling, meaning no one other than yourself can know precisely how you are feeling it. This means no two people will experience pain in the same way: the exact same finger prick may be perceived quite differently by two different people. An injured person can even be initially unaware of his injury because he does not feel it at first. Probably you have experienced a situation in which, distracted by something else, you did not feel a stubbed toe or a bug bite to the same extent you would have if your mind were not focused on something else.

This variability in how pain is perceived is because the simple electrical signal running up your finger from that needle prick gets modulated by a maze of other nerve cells in the spinal cord and in the brain. Some of these influences dampen down the signal, others ramp it up. The result is that when it finally gets to your upper brain, where your consciousness lies, all sorts of things have affected the signal, things that are unique to you and your brain.

You have several kinds of nerve fibers in your finger. The ones that transmit the fastest signals, the heavily myelinated ones, mostly are concerned with light touch and position sense, which is knowing where your finger is in space. This makes sense, because these bits of information are things the brain needs to learn as rapidly as possible. If you want to demonstrate this for yourself, close your eyes, open your mouth, and rapidly stick your finger in your mouth. You can do this without poking yourself in the eye because your brain knows, every millisecond, just where your finger is in space in relation to your mouth. These nerves are also involved in the pain response, particularly in blocking some of its input in the spinal cord. When they do not work, the perceived pain from a pricked finger is worse.

The nerve fibers in your finger that transmit pain signals, the ones with less or no myelin insulation, can sense three kinds of things: mechanical forces like hard pressure, hot and cold, and chemical substances. If you pay attention when you whack your finger with a hammer, hard as that may be to do, you can distinguish between both types of nerve fibers in action. You first feel a very sharp, very localized pain. This is a signal from the insulated fibers, which gets to your brain first. An instant later you begin to feel a more diffuse, deeper pain that is less well localized to the precise spot. This is input from the slower fibers with no myelin.

Another way we experience the difference between fast and slow fibers is when we bump our shin on a piece of furniture when walking in the dark. We first feel our leg hit the furniture—those are the insulated touch and position sense fibers at work. After a perceptible lag, we feel like yowling in pain—those are the uninsulated pain fibers catching up with their messages.

Stimulating one set of fibers, particularly the fast, insulated ones, affects how our brain processes these sensations. Every parent knows how to do this, although you probably did not know why it works. When your child comes running to you after falling down and bonking her head, what do you do? Generally you rub it, and it really does feel better. This is not just from parental love. Stimulating the touch fibers in the same place where the pain is coming from causes them to intervene and dampen the pain signal coming from the other fibers. The same thing happens when we rub any body part after hitting it on something.

In your son's infected finger, the nerves that are causing him pain are the chemical receptors. All those inflammatory substances the macrophages and phagocytes released did more than make the capillary blood vessels leak and summon other cellular soldiers to the area. They also stimulated his nerve endings, instructing them to send a message of pain up the electrical grid to his spinal cord and then on to his brain.

Your daughter's appendicitis pain was of a different sort. The nerve fibers in the intestines are not sensitive to being stuck with a sharp needle or being touched. What they are sensitive to is being stretched, as anybody who has ever had severe gas pains can testify. When her appendix first started getting inflamed, that is what happened: things were being stretched. As matters progressed, however, she got a different kind of pain—a sharp, localized pain in the lower right side of her abdomen. That was because the process had begun to inflame the lining of her abdomen, and that region is richly supplied with nerve fibers that are more like those in the finger.

There are other places besides the intestines where stretching and pressure are the main pain-causing signals. The middle ear is one of these, which is one reason your son's ear hurt when he had an infection there: the pressure from all the fluid in that tiny space caused pressure. His eardrum was red and inflamed as well, and that also contributed to his misery by stimulating pain fibers there.

Now that you have some understanding of where pain comes from, you can understand how the medicines that we use to treat it work. We have two main approaches for treating pain: we can do things that reduce the pain signals coming from the spot that hurts, or we can use medications that confuse the brain into thinking the pain is either not there or is not so bad.

You saw an example of how the first method works in the scenario with your son's finger. After you soaked it in warm water, the infected area opened and spontaneously drained out a good measure of the infected soup of bacteria and phagocytes. That both relieved some of the pressure on the mechanical nerve receptors and removed a lot of the materials that were triggering the chemical receptors.

There are other things we can do to reduce the pain signals. Cooling the area with an ice pack is one way. Another is to put a medicine on the spot that interferes with how the nerves work. Examples of this approach include eardrops that can numb the eardrum of a child with an infection or numbing sprays and ointments for a child with sunburn. A dentist injecting a painkiller around a sore tooth is using a more powerful version of these same methods.

The other way to treat pain is to use medications that act directly on the nervous system to alter how the brain reacts to the signals coming from the painful place. They convince the brain to downplay or even ignore the information. This is how both acetaminophen (Tylenol and many other brands) and ibuprofen (Motrin and many other brands) work. Ibuprofen also relieves pain in another way that acetaminophen does not: ibuprofen can work directly at the site, such as the inflamed finger or ear, to block the production of some of those substances that cause the inflammation. We also have an injectable medication related to ibuprofen, only more potent, called ketorolac (brand name Toradol).

More severe pain calls for medications more powerful than these. Members of the opiate family, also called narcotics, are the standard. There are many members of this family, which vary in how they are given, their appropriate dose, and some of their side effects, but they all work in the same way: they go to the brain and the spinal cord and alter a person's perception of the pain. They also can alter mood and a person's level of awareness to things around them. A common oral narcotic used for children is codeine; a common injectable one is morphine.

Even though we give narcotic medications for severe pain, a fascinating thing about them is that they are not really foreign to the body at all. We have similar substances that occur naturally in our body, and presumably these natural narcotics are performing some useful function inside us, most likely involving pain control. So when we give a child with more severe pain, such as a broken leg, a medication of this type, we are really just reinforcing a normal pathway. The presence of these natural substances could explain why some people, an Indian Yogi for example, can walk across a bed of hot coals without pain, because he has learned to alter his brain's perception of what is painful.

Pain, uncomfortable as it is, does serve some useful purpose, and in that sense helps a child heal. Pain alerts us that something is wrong and tells us we should try to do something about it. If we cannot feel the pain, worse injury often results. A good example of this is when a person lacks sensation in an arm or a leg: because he cannot feel pain there, painful things, such as an ill-fitting shoe, can go unnoticed and lead to injury.

But pain can also interfere with healing. Mild or moderate pain does not seem to affect healing much, but more severe pain, if it persists, can interfere with healing. This stems from the effects of what we call stress hormones, substances like adrenaline, which the body releases at times of stress. They are called "fight or flight" hormones because they probably helped our ancient ancestors deal with things like wild animal attacks. Although they can help in times of acute danger, prolonged high levels of these hormones, such as with continuing severe pain, do inhibit proper healing. Researchers have studied this phenomenon in children who have had major surgery, and it is clear that using painkillers does not just make the children feel better—it also makes them heal better.

FEVER

Fever means an abnormal elevation of body temperature. But what is abnormal? Most of us have heard or read that "normal" is 98.6° Fahrenheit, which is 37° centigrade. In fact, normal temperature varies throughout the day. It is as much as one degree lower in the morning than in the afternoon, and exertion of any kind raises it. Where you measure it also matters. Internal temperature, such as taken on a child with a rectal thermometer, is usually a degree or so higher than a simultaneous measurement taken in the mouth or under the armpit.

There is also a range of what is normal for each individual—not all people are the same. So what is a fever in me may not be a fever in you. As a practical matter, most doctors stay clear of this controversy by choosing a number that is high enough so that individual variability does not matter. Most choose a value of 100.4° Fahrenheit, or 38° centigrade as the definition of fever. It is not a perfect answer, but it is a number that has stood the test of time in practice.

We maintain our normal body temperature in several ways. Chief among them is our blood circulation. Heat radiates from our body surface, so by directing blood toward or away from our skin we can unload or conserve heat. We can also control body temperature by sweating—evaporation of sweat cools us down. We know how important a mechanism this is because the rare person who cannot sweat or who is taking a medicine that interferes with sweating has trouble keeping his body temperature regulated when he gets sick. If a swing in blood flow inward to raise temperature happens very fast, we respond by shivering. This is also why we shiver if we go outside without a coat in the winter; our bodies are redirecting blood flow from our skin to our core in order to maintain temperature.

All parents know that a common cause of fever in children is infection. A more precise way to think about it is that a common cause of fever is your old friend inflammation. Because infection is the most common cause of inflammation in children, we generally assume a child with a fever has an infection somewhere in her body unless we can prove otherwise.

Our brains have a kind of thermostat built into them. Like the thermostat in a house, it senses the temperature of the blood passing by it and uses a series of controlling valves in the blood circulation to fine-tune the temperature. Also like your house thermostat, it continues to sense the temperature and adjust it as necessary until it has reached the value for which the thermostat is set. Fever happens when the thermostat is reset, just as when you twist the dial on the wall for your furnace—the body reacts to bring itself to the new setting. What twists the knob on the brain's thermostat to cause fever are substances in the blood.

These fever-inducing substances belong to the same familiar family of inflammatory molecules you encountered in your child's finger, ear, and appendix. Mostly they come from macrophages, but germs themselves can also release things that have the same effect. The sudden rises and falls parents often see in their child's temperature when she has an infection reflect the usually brief time these substances are in the blood. Sustained fever for many hours can happen if these materials are steadily present.

Opinions vary among doctors about when fever needs treatment. Fever itself virtually never causes harm on its own. The only times it can do harm is when it gets very, very high—106° or more—for a sustained period. That only happens in highly unusual situations; ordinary childhood infections never get that high. It is true fever can make a child uncomfortable, although children generally tolerate it much better than adults. For that reason alone, many doctors advise treatment.

There is another reason to treat fever. Toddlers may experience brief convulsions—seizures—when their body temperature rises very fast. These so-called febrile seizures cause no harm to the brain itself and often run in families, but fever treatment makes good sense for a child who has had them in the past.

We have two effective drugs to treat fever, the same acetaminophen and ibuprofen you read about in the section on pain. Both work the same way: they reset the brain thermostat to a lower lever. Both only last a few of hours or so in their effect, which is why you will see your child's fever go back up again when they wear off if there are still any of those fever-causing substances from the inflamed site still in the circulation.

NAUSEA, RETCHING, AND VOMITING

Most of us are familiar with nausea, that queasy feeling experience has taught us may soon be followed by vomiting. When that happens, we begin to feel a quiver at the base of our tongue and in the back of our throat. At this point we may be able to suppress the feeling enough to keep from vomiting by swallowing a few times or taking some deep breaths. If none of that works, we soon expel whatever is inside our stomach out through our mouths, after which the nausea is typically improved, at least for a short time. If there is nothing in our stomachs, we may still go through the vomiting reflex—the dry heaves.

Vomiting differs from mere spitting up, what parents of a baby often call a "wet burp." Vomiting is a very forceful act involving contraction of powerful muscles in the stomach and abdomen. When a baby spits up, it is because the muscular tissue at the junction between her stomach and the lower part of her esophagus is too lax to keep the food inside. We call that regurgitation or reflux of stomach contents. An older child or adult with heartburn is experiencing a version of the same thing, except the stomach contents usually do not make it all the way up into the mouth. Spitting up is simply a local event in the lower esophagus, with the stomach contents running back up the wrong way for a moment. In contrast, vomiting is a complex reflex in which several parts of the brain and the digestive system need to communicate with each other and coordinate what they are doing.

Both nausea and vomiting are controlled by a place in the lower part of the brain in the region we call the brain stem. Regulatory centers for many of our basic reflexes, like the one that keeps us breathing, are located nearby. This fact tells us that vomiting is an ancient and primitive reflex that has been with us for a very long time. Doctors are notorious for devising esoteric and fancy names for anatomic places, but this spot in the brain is called by a very practical term—the vomiting center.

Many things can awaken the vomiting center and cause it to do its job. Signals from the higher centers in the brain where we do our thinking can do it. Anyone who has had a queasy thought after seeing something distasteful can attest to this connection. The links between the vomiting center and the parts of the brain that regulate balance are especially close, which is why a ride in a roller coaster or a bumpy airplane can make you throw up. The vomiting center also is sensitive to mechanical pressure on it, so vomiting is a common symptom when people have increased pressure inside their brain.

The vomiting center also quickly responds to a whole host of things it detects in the bloodstream. Many medications have nausea and vomiting as a side effect. This is a particular problem with some of the drugs we use to treat cancer. We even have drugs we can give to induce vomiting as their intended effect. Changes in the body's hormones, such as occurs with pregnancy, can activate the center. The majority of women will have at least some problems with nausea and vomiting when they are pregnant, especially during the early months.

For a parent with a sick child, the most important things that tickle the vomiting center are those that happen in the digestive tract, since many disorders of the stomach and intestines lead to vomiting. There are nerves located throughout the digestive tract, especially in the upper portions of it, which run back to the vomiting center. These even begin in the mouth, which is why a person who gags when the back of the throat is touched may quickly vomit. For some people, even brushing their teeth can bring this on if they are not careful.

For the stomach and small intestines, any inflammation there sends messages back up the neural network to the vomiting center. If the signals are strong enough, the person will vomit. For children, the most common cause of this is a viral infection, the stomach flu. You read in the section about pain that intestinal nerves are especially sensitive to stretching. This also applies to the nerves that control nausea and vomiting, so a digestive tract that is stretched full of air and food that is not going anywhere can do more than hurt: it is also primed for the vomiting reflex. We know this is so because, in such a situation, often the simple technique of slipping a tube down into the stagnant lake of stuff in the stomach and upper intestines and sucking it out will relieve a person's nausea and vomiting.

The vomiting act itself, though it happens quickly, is an intricate series of events. When the vomiting center sends out the "go" signal, the stomach muscles first relax, halting any further movement of its contents. The next stage is what is properly called retching, which is several sharp, jerky spasms of the muscles in the chest and of the diaphragm, the powerful muscle sheet that spans the floor of the chest and separates the heart and lungs from the stomach, intestines, and other organs in the abdomen. Part of the retching reflex is to close the vocal cords tightly together. Then comes the actual vomiting. The abdominal muscles squeeze the stomach, the esophagus opens, and whatever is in the stomach comes back out. The vocal cords stay shut, preventing any of the vomited material from getting into the lungs. This is an important protective reflex; when it malfunctions, stomach contents with all their acid can cause serious injury to the lungs.

We know a lot about what things trigger the vomiting center and how they do it. The particular molecular signals themselves are even known. This information has allowed researchers to fashion drugs that block these signals. These drugs are most effective for the vomiting caused by extremely powerful signals to the vomiting center, such as those that come from cancer treatment drugs. A drug called ondansetron (brand name Zofran) is an example.

Most parents deal with vomiting children in the context of the stomach flu. For these children, whose vomiting is less severe, doctors generally do not recommend using any of the drugs that suppress the vomiting center. There are several good reasons for this recommendation. The antivomiting drugs work on the brain by blocking the action of several molecules that brain cells use to talk to one another, called neurotransmitters. The drugs target neurotransmitters that are particularly abundant in the vomiting center. But these neurotransmitters work elsewhere in the brain, too, and blocking them can cause unwanted side effects, especially in children. There are exceptions to everything in medicine, but since the vomiting from stomach flu is not severe and passes in a day or so, the risk of side effects from these medications generally outweighs the potential benefit of using them.

Is vomiting of any use, and does it help healing when your child is sick? Certainly it is helpful for the body to have a way to get unwanted and toxic material quickly out of the digestive system, and vomiting accomplishes that. Nausea seems a useful thing to have, too, as a way of notifying us that vomiting is likely to follow.

Until recently doctors deliberately provoked vomiting in children who had eaten something potentially dangerous, and we advised parents to keep ipecac, a drug that does this, handy for such an occasion. We no longer recommend this because the risk of all the retching and throwing up outweighs any benefit. For parents, it is logical to regard vomiting as a natural reflex that may be doing some good, in spite of the brief misery it can cause a child. Because the drugs that either block or provoke vomiting can have significant side effects, in nearly all situations, it is best to let nature decide when she is going to make use of the reflex.

DIARRHEA

Diarrhea, the frequent passage of watery stools, is something with which most parents of small children are well acquainted. It is a common symptom, because its most common causes, intestinal viruses, are all around us. There are many of these for a child's immune system to meet as it matures. Each new encounter usually causes illness, but subsequent exposures often cause few or no problems. These viruses are highly infectious, so they spread easily wherever toddlers gather to share toys and food. The result is what doctors call gastroenteritis, a fancy term for an inflamed stomach and intestines.

Other things besides viruses can cause diarrhea, such as celiac disease that you learned about in the last chapter, but most of these cause it in the same way—injuring the cells lining the intestines so they cannot do their job of absorbing the nutrients passing by them. A wide variety of food intolerances can also lead to diarrhea, often because the absorbing cells, though present in the intestine, are unable to deal with a particular food properly in some individuals. Common examples of this include a deficiency of the absorbing cells that process lactose, a type of sugar in dairy products, or a sensitivity to the proteins present in cow's milk. Whatever the cause of the poor functioning of the absorbing cell lining, the result is often diarrhea. If there is significant stretching and squeezing going on in the intestine, the child will often have cramping pain, too.

When the intestinal lining is injured, it cannot do its job of absorbing food. If a large amount of unabsorbed food makes it to the lower reaches of the small intestine, it draws water out of the intestinal wall. It also becomes excellent food for all the bacteria living there, and the action of the germs gorging themselves on this sudden feast produces even more substances that draw water into the intestine. When this mixture is dumped into the large intestine, the enormous mass of bacteria normally living there magnifies the effect. The large intestine can absorb quite a bit of water, but it can become overwhelmed by the volume. Plus, its lining cells may themselves be injured by the infection, making them less able to do their job.

These things make the stools watery. Diarrhea also means more frequent stools. The simple increase in the amount of material the colon must deal with is one cause of the more frequent stools. Another is that most causes of diarrhea also speed up the transit time, the length of time it takes for what is swallowed to pass all the way through.

There is another kind of diarrhea, one less common in children. This disorder is of the large intestine, the colon, and is called colitis, because that word means "inflamed colon." It is typically caused by one of several varieties of infectious bacteria. Since the colon can become quite irritated and inflamed, the diarrhea of colitis often has blood in it that oozed off the intestinal wall. It is usually a more serious illness than simple gastroenteritis of the upper reaches of the intestine. This is why seeing blood in your child's stools is a reason to visit or call the doctor, especially if your child has fever as well.

We have several ways of dealing with diarrhea, the first of which is to do nothing other than to ensure your child is getting enough fluid to replace that lost in the stools. This is how doctors usually handle the situation, because typical gastroenteritis is quite self-limited and passes soon. When it does, the damaged absorbing cells very rapidly replace themselves on the villi, and all is well. If it persists for many days, as it did in your nephew with celiac disease, there is reason to suspect something else is causing it.

Simple common sense teaches us we should not challenge the intestines of a child with diarrhea with large meals full of complex, difficult to absorb foods, because the poorer the absorption, the worse the diarrhea potential. Parents have known this for generations. This is the rationale for using smaller, more frequent meals of simple starches like rice and bread or even of eliminating all solids for a day or so. There are several ways of approaching this issue, but many parents find out by trial and error which dietary manipulations work for their children and which ones do not.

We do have several drugs to treat diarrhea, most of which work by slowing down the transit time through the intestines. Lomotil is the brand name of a commonly used one. These drugs affect the intestinal nerves that control how fast the intestines squeeze the food along, slowing down the process. They work well in adults, although you can easily see how it is possible to overshoot and end up with constipation. However, doctors rarely recommend these drugs for small children because—as with the nausea and vomiting medicines—the potential side effects outweigh any benefit of using them for a condition that usually quickly passes without treatment.

COUGH

The hallmark of most respiratory illness, both in children and in adults, is a cough. The trip you took into your son's lungs puts you in an excellent position to know just why this is so. Coughing is a reflex, one difficult to suppress. You probably know this from the experience of sitting in a quiet setting, such as in a lecture audience or in church, when you have a cold. The urge to cough is nearly impossible to deny, even with intense effort.

The upper and middle portions of the airway, meaning the space between the back of the throat, through the vocal cords, and down to the first branching of the windpipe, are thickly sown with sensors. They are particularly abundant right around the vocal cords and down at the area of the first branching. If anything touches these sensors, the response is a cough. The reason this reflex is so powerful is that nature is fanatic about protecting our airways. We need to breathe every minute, and objects that might block our airways are potentially very dangerous. Since the last line of defense for the lungs is at the first branching of the windpipe, it makes sense that touching that spot provokes a particularly explosive episode of coughing.

Infections of the upper respiratory tract cause the mucous-secreting cells that line the walls to make more mucus, sometimes large amounts of it, and this extra material trips the cough sensors. The upshot is that we cough and cough until the mucus is cleared from the airway via a mechanism doctors term a "productive cough," meaning it produces sputum.

Often, however, a cough is dry—it does not produce any sputum at all because the cause for it is not excess mucus. We term this a nonproductive cough. It often comes in spasms of multiple coughs in succession, followed by a period of relative quiet. This kind of cough is caused by inflammation of the walls of the airway, something respiratory viruses do, and the inflammation triggers the cough sensors. In children, asthma is another common cause, because asthma inflames the airways. A nonproductive cough can also happen if we inhale anything that irritates our airways, such as dust, smoke, or a noxious gas.

There are dozens of over-the-counter products sold as remedies for cough. None of them do much to help it, although they may soothe the back of the throat. The ingredients many of them contain cause unwanted side effects in small children, so most doctors do not recommend using them, nor does the American Academy of Pediatrics. The last thing we want in a medication for children is something that does not help the situation and may actually cause harm.

We have medicines that really do suppress cough. They do not work on the airway; rather, they work on the brain itself to suppress the cough reflex. Codeine, a narcotic, is the one most commonly used, but there are others. We rarely use these medicines in children, especially small children, because they have significant side effects, primarily drowsiness and altered mental state. Additionally, if a cough is being caused by excess mucus or other material in the airway, we can make the situation worse by blocking the child's ability to clear the stuff out.

ITCHING

Itching is a common symptom when children get a rash from any cause. You read in the last chapter about poison ivy, for example, which produces intense itching. I include itching in this chapter, but you have already seen all you need to know about its causes in your explorations of the last chapter. The mast cells in the skin are coated with the special antibody immunoglobulin E and are stuffed full of histamine. As you read, they release their histamine when stimulated. The histamine has an immediate effect on the meshwork of tiny nerve fibers in the skin, sending signals up to the spinal cord and further on to the brain. The result is the sensation we know as an itch.

Although allergies and histamine are among the strongest triggers for itching, there are others. Any sort of inflammation in the skin, with its array of molecular signals and messages the cells use to communicate and call for help can set off the itch nerves. This is why many childhood rashes itch. Even the substances cells use to talk back and forth as they heal a previously damaged area can trigger the feeling, which is why it is common to feel itching in a newly forming scar.

You read in the section about pain how rubbing a painful spot can briefly tone down the pain signals coming up the nerve network. Itching is an example of the same thing. When we scratch an itch, the sensory stimulus of the scratch momentarily wipes out the signal from the nerves sending the itch message. We all know that the relief is only temporary; the itch often returns, worse than it was before we gave in to the urge to scratch.

This phenomenon is called the "itch-scratch cycle" by dermatologists, the skin specialists. The scratching causes further inflammation of the skin, which causes worse itching, which leads to more scratching, and so on until skin can become quite damaged. The urge to itch is a powerful one. It can make concentrating on anything else or sleep impossible. Fortunately, we have several ways to treat itching.

Treating symptoms can make your child feel better, but, as you have read, in most common situations, treating symptoms does not really speed physical healing. (Psychological healing is another matter, as you will read later.) Itching is different, because breaking the itch-scratch cycle helps the skin heal. It also can prevent a complication of scratching: fingernails can carry skin bacteria beneath the skin, bypassing the normal barrier, and cause a secondary infection in the skin.

We have two ways of treating itching. We can do things to the place that itches to soothe the inflammation and thus dampen the itch signal going up the nerves. This can be something simple, as in the case of itchy, dry skin that needs only moisturizing lotion to get the job done. A variety of soothing lotions and baths can accomplish the same thing in a child with a rash. We also can use creams that suppress the inflammation in the skin. Hydrocortisone cream (with its many steroid relatives) does this, although it takes a day or so to begin working. These medications should not be used for prolonged periods, especially on the face, but they can break the self-perpetuating itch-scratch cycle. Finally, we can use one of the medicines you read about in the chapter on allergies that block the effects of histamine. These usually help, but because not all the itch signals are from histamine, antihistamines do not eliminate them.

MALAISE

We end this chapter with the most nonspecific symptom of all, what doctors call malaise—that vague feeling of unwellness that often is the very first symptom of any illness. It is listlessness, a sense that something is not quite right inside. Often it makes us feel achy all over without localizing to any particular spot. Adults find it hard to describe, and it is even more difficult for a child to express what he is feeling. A parent can usually spot it in her child, though, and knows that it means other symptoms are to follow.

Malaise is bodywide evidence that somewhere those cellular mediators—the messages that cells use both to do their work and to summon help to a site of inflammation or infection—have made it into the bloodstream and are circulating around. Often the next phase is fever, since some of these substances reset the brain thermostat, but body temperature need not change for a person to feel the symptom. Malaise is frustratingly imprecise as a symptom, but nearly all of us know it when we feel it. The body might control whatever that is, leaving us feeling fine the next day, but it might not, in which case the problem will have declared itself by then.

· 8 ·

How Injuries Heal: An Inside Expedition to Bruises and Broken Bones

$\mathcal{A}$ child's body faces other challenges besides dealing with germs, ragweed pollen, and poison ivy. Children also get a lot of scrapes, lumps, and bumps. These things need to heal, too, and they nearly always do. This chapter is about how that happens.

This chapter's scenario again stars your handyman son, he of the infected finger in chapter 1. He is back to building things, and this time he has decided to build a tree house in the backyard. Had he shared his plans with you, you probably would not have given him the go-ahead to do it, because the branches of this particular tree are many feet above the ground.

Your first inkling of what he was up to came in the form of his cry from the yard. When you hustle outside to see what is wrong, you discover he has fallen from one of the higher limbs. He landed on his outstretched left hand, and you can easily see it is bent at a crazy angle just above his wrist. He clearly has a broken arm, a fracture.

He seems okay otherwise. The arm hurts, of course, but curiously not as much as you would think. As you read in the last chapter, this is often the case immediately after an injury. Looking at it makes you a little queasy. Also after reading the last chapter, you know how this works; neural connections from the thinking part of your brain run straight to your vomiting center, waking it and getting it ready to do its job. But you do not throw up. Purposeful activity often can lull the vomiting center back to sleep, such as when you run back into the house to get some towels and pillows to cradle and cushion his arm. You load him into the car, and the two of you head for the hospital emergency department.

When you get to the hospital, the staff moves you to the front of the waiting line. They are well acquainted with active children with broken arms. The emergency department physician looks your son over quickly, asks you a few simple questions about his general state of health, and then tells the nurses to place an intravenous line—a tiny plastic tube that goes into a vein on his good hand, through which he can receive fluids and medications.

By this time his arm really has begun to hurt, so the staff gives him a dose of morphine, one of the stronger painkillers you read about. It works very well for situations like this. Within a few minutes he feels better, because the morphine has reached deep into his nervous system and adjusted the signals coming up from the nerves around the injury. His lower arm and wrist still ache, but the sharp, stabbing pains are gone. He is able to sit on the emergency department cart and rest his arm on a large pillow.

A short time later an orthopedic surgeon, a broken bone expert, arrives to look at your son. He gingerly examines the broken part, but does not move it around too much. He pays particular attention to your son's hand and fingers beyond the break, looking to see that his fingers are pink and that he has a normal sense of touch, which he does. This is important information for the doctor: the wrist is a small space, and bundles of nerves and blood vessels run through it on their way to the hand. The doctor needs to know right away if the fracture has affected any of these important structures.

Preliminaries done, the doctor sends you and your son down the hall to the radiology department to get an x-ray of the fracture. This might seem unnecessary to some parents. After all, the arm is clearly broken. Why would we need an x-ray to verify the obvious? The reason is that the precise nature of the fracture affects how the orthopedist deals with it.

There are several general classifications of fractures: a closed, or simple, fracture means the ends of the broken bones are sealed beneath the skin; a comminuted fracture describes one in which the bone is broken into several pieces; an open, or compound, fracture is one in which you can see part of the bone through a break in the skin. Your son clearly does not have a compound fracture, but in order to fix your son's arm, the orthopedist needs to know the details of how the broken ends of the bones relate to each other. Since a single x-ray gives only a two-dimensional picture, he usually needs several views taken from different angles.

Once you two are back from radiology, the doctor is ready to fix the arm. He will do what we call a closed reduction of the fracture, commonly called "bone setting" during our great-grandparents' era. We have two bones in our forearm: the radius is on the thumb side, the ulna is on the pinky finger side. Your son broke both of them, a common event when a person falls on an outstretched hand. Both need to be fixed.

As you would expect, reducing a fracture like this—pulling the edges back together and straightening his arm out—really hurts. The morphine your son got controls the pain as long as nobody is pulling on his arm, but it will not be enough to get him through the reduction procedure. He will need a more powerful sedative drug given through his vein to help the morphine. Using those medications safely requires that a child have an empty stomach, which your son fortunately has, since it is now midafternoon, and he has had nothing to eat since an early breakfast. Even with the sedative in his system, the moment the orthopedist pulls on the wrist would be painful without something else to help, so the doctor injects a medication directly around the broken edges of the bones to numb all the nerves there.

Your son is now ready to get a closed reduction of his fracture. The doctor asks you if you want to stay and watch or go outside and wait. You decide to stay—sitting down, just in case. Your son is lying on his back, appropriately groggy and snoozing from morphine and sedatives, and the area around the broken edges of bone is nicely numb. He looks comfortable. The doctor picks up the broken arm below the elbow and suspends it in the air by hooking your son's fingers to a pole next to the bed by gently fastening his fingers to an array of wires on the pole. Using a quick motion, he straightens the arm. He then fashions a fiberglass cast to hold the ends in place. Another x-ray then verifies the bone ends are where the doctor wants them to be. Your son awakens from his nap, and the two of you go home. The tree house project will have to wait.

The bones are special places in the body, with their own specialized structures and architecture. Most of us have 206 of them in total. They are the scaffold that holds us up—without them we would collapse like gelatin. Some of them also protect vital organs, as the skull encloses and shields the brain. We tend to think of bones as inert struts and girders, but they are far from that. A child's bones are as alive, busy, and active as any other system in his body.

To understand what is going on in bones and thus how your son's arm heals, you need to go in and have a close look. As in our previous scenarios, before you can appreciate how a fracture heals, you need first to visit a normal bone. In your past adventures you were forced to cast yourself back in time and explore the body before anything happened. In this scenario you do not have to do that. You can combine everything into one trip by first exploring his unbroken right arm and then proceeding over to the injured one. The best time to take this trip is after your son has gotten the morphine, so he is comfortable and it is safe to leave him for a little while, and before the orthopedist has fixed the fracture. Imagine you are doing it while everyone is waiting for the first set of x-rays to be processed.

You now know several ways you can get inside his body. Any of these will get you to the bloodstream highway you need to reach his arm. His nose is the closest, so you choose it. Once inside, you dive down through the mucous layer, wriggle between the phalanx of lining cells, and look around for a handy capillary vessel. Which one you choose does not matter, since you can follow any of them downstream, gaining new tributaries as you go. These coalesce to form first small veins, then larger ones, and you soon find yourself in one of the largest veins in the body, called the superior vena cava. It plugs directly into the heart. You next flash through what is called the right side of the heart and then rocket back out toward the lungs, riding along in the pulmonary artery, the huge conduit that takes blood from the right side of the heart out to the lungs to pick up oxygen.

You have been in this region before, during your son's asthma attack. Except last time you were on the other side of things; you were inside an air sac looking at the blood streaming around you in the walls. Now you are part of that stream. You are past the air sacs in an instant, noticing as you pass that the red blood cells all around you have changed their hue from a darker to a brighter red as they take on oxygen. Then you are back in the heart again, only this time on the left side.

This pumping chamber shoots you out the aorta, the principal blood vessel carrying oxygenated blood to the body. It is a fast ride because the velocity of the bloodstream at this spot is enormous. You have to maneuver and think fast because the aorta quickly sends off tributaries, called the great vessels, and you need to take the very first one of these to get to his right arm, the uninjured one. If you stayed in the middle of the stream you would end up in his legs. Once inside the first artery branching off the aorta, you immediately swerve again to avoid being sent out the vessel leading to his head. Your way is straight along toward his arm. You are soon in his radial artery, the one you can easily feel making the pulse in your wrist near the thumb. You dart off into a small tributary that takes you to your destination—his radius, one of the bones that is broken in his other arm.

You are approaching the surface of the bone through a small blood vessel that looks as if it will soon dive right down into the bone substance. You do not want to do that quite yet; you want to have a look around at the outside of the bone, so you snag a spot on the vessel wall and worm your way between the lining cells until you are out of it and into the surrounding tissues. You are soon crawling on the surface of the bone itself.

You see that the bone is covered by a kind of quilt, a lush membrane that has a large number of capillary blood vessels running in it. This is called the periosteum. As you pass through it, you see it has a couple of layers, and one of these is heavily populated with cells of a sort you have never seen before. These are primitive bone cells, something unique to bone. Think of them as a reserve of future bone cells, waiting in their embryonic state until they are needed. When they are, they quickly mature into ordinary bone cells and go about making new bone. Meanwhile they wait patiently until called.

After you have passed through the periosteum you find yourself parked on the actual bone itself. You are not surprised to find it is white and it is hard, just as you think bone should be. You are surprised, however, that it is not an entirely solid, impenetrable surface. All around you are tiny holes, through which a multitude of small blood vessels bore their way inside the bone. You are resting on what we call cortical bone. If you had a drill, you could buzz your way through it like a hard rock miner, but you do not, so the only way inside is to travel within one of those blood vessels.

Once you are through the surface, you see that the bone is not as solid as it first appears to be. The cortical bone is only a quarter inch or so thick. It forms a hard shell around what, at your present size, looks like a crazy maze of struts and girders running every which way. This region is called spongy bone and is found mostly near the ends of the long bones such as the arms and legs.

You can tell this is a very busy place, especially at the end of his arm bone where you are. Since your son is a growing boy, the regions at the ends of his bones are continually laying down new bone. These busy cellular carpenters first construct bands of fibers that look much like the connective tissue you have seen in other places. But then they do something quite different to it: they use a mixture of minerals—calcium and phosphate salts—to make these connective tissue bands solid and hard, like gypsum dry wall. Depending upon how hard the cells want the resulting bone to be, they can fashion the softer girders of spongy bone or the harder ones of cortical bone.

As you pick your way through the maze of beams you see, off in a corner, another kind of cell. This one is bigger than the carpenter cells, and it seems to be doing an extraordinary thing—it is methodically tearing up the structures that the other cells have built. It is working right next to a construction gang, which seems to be totally ignoring the vandalism going on nearby. Why would the body do such a thing? It appears to make no sense. It is like hiring one person to dig holes and another to fill them in.

In fact, the delicate balance between building and taking apart is crucial to how bones do their job. Bones are like homeowners who are never quite happy with their houses and for that reason are forever remodeling. That is indeed what we call it—bone remodeling. Bones are continually fine-tuning their structure because the demands put upon them are ever changing. Changes in how we bear weight on our bones and what we do with them—such as how much and what kind of exercise we do—cause them to remodel themselves in ways designed to do their job better. In a child, whose bones are growing, the activities of building far overshadow those of tearing down, but some remodeling happens.

You turn your attention from the cellular construction crew and look at what else is around you. Here you see more evidence that any notions we might have of bones being a boring backwater of the body are wrong. There is busyness everywhere. You are at the edge of the bone marrow, the sheltered area inside the bones where blood cells are made. Macrophages and mast cells are made there, too. Not all bones participate in this equally; in adults, most blood cells are made in the flat bones like the pelvic bones and the breastbone. In young children, however, the long bones like the arm bone you are presently in also contribute.

If you look with the naked eye at a full-size, opened long bone, you can distinguish between two kinds of marrow, called red marrow and yellow marrow. The red marrow is where blood cells are made, which is why it is red; the yellow marrow is made yellow from fat cells. In babies, nearly all marrow is red marrow. By adulthood, most of the cavities inside long bones are made up of yellow marrow. Children like your son are somewhere in between.

The red marrow is the factory where all those phagocytes you have seen during your travels to various places around the body are made. It is a factory that can ramp up production extremely fast when needed. In the infected finger you saw legions of phagocytes arrive to fight the germs. These first responders were already on duty, and they could react nearly immediately when they were called. But after a few hours, the first phagocytes were done for, having sacrificed themselves in the fight. All the later ones came from the switched-on production facility of the bone marrow.

When things are quiet a phagocyte lives for several days after leaving the bone marrow. It spends a few hours in the circulation before moving out of it in search of something to destroy. In contrast, when the body's need is high, the time elapsed between a phagocyte leaving the marrow and being consumed in an inflammation war is often a matter of a few hours or even less. The marrow normally makes more than a billion of these cells each day. When needed, the marrow can churn out many times that number.

The marrow also makes red blood cells, the specialized cell that does only one thing—haul oxygen from the lungs and deliver it all around the body. Red cells live considerably longer than phagocytes, typically several months, and they normally do not leave the bloodstream. In spite of their longevity, the marrow still must make several million of them each second to replace worn-out ones.

If that were not enough to do, the marrow factory also makes a tiny bit of a thing called a blood platelet. Platelets are not really cells. Rather, they are buds that shed off a specialized factory cell in the marrow and then go out into the bloodstream. Platelets are crucial to making blood clot properly. As you will see, they are also key players in the drama of tissue healing anywhere blood has formed clots.

Your son's arm bone is a hustling, bustling place. It is intriguing that nature stuck the process of manufacturing blood cells inside the bones, since on the face of it, making blood cells has nothing to do with the supporting scaffold function of our skeletons. Doing it that way does protect the cellular machinery, but it seems as if nature is making use of a handy, otherwise empty spare room in the body to house this vital activity.

Now you have seen the inner secrets of a typical long bone in a child. It is hard to imagine just what would happen if this snug cavern inside its protective hard shell were snapped open, spilling its contents out. Is it like a major earthquake, one that takes down buildings and rips up concrete highways? How can such a thing heal? To find out, you must turn around and travel over to your son's other arm. There is still time, since the orthopedist will not be fixing the fracture for another hour or so.

The best way for you to get a good look at what is happening there is to pick a tributary blood vessel halfway down his injured forearm and follow it to a stretch of healthy bone. Then you can crawl your vehicle along the periosteal covering until you get to the action. Before you reach it, though, you find yourself approaching what looks like a big mass of red gelatin. When you arrive at the edge of this blob, you see it is made of uncountable numbers of red blood cells, roped all around and trapped in what resembles an enormous spider's web. Long strands of the webbing run in all directions and are linked together in many spots to create a meshwork with holes so small the red blood cells are snagged inside it.

You are looking at a huge blood clot. When your son's bones broke, the rich collection of blood vessels on the periosteum covering the bone— as well as some inside the bone—broke, too. These severed vessels spilled their contents into the space between and around the broken ends of the bone. Within minutes this liquid blood congealed into the morass you now see. The clot serves as a patch in the blood vessels, blocking off any further bleeding. That is its immediate purpose. But the blood-clotting system also plays a crucial role in the drama of tissue healing after injuries such as this one.

Microscopic organisms, like bacteria, can absorb what they need to live directly from the environment around them. As soon as creatures appeared that have more than a few layers of cells between their insides and their outsides, there had to be a way to transport these essential materials to the cells living deep below the surface. As organisms became still more complex, there also needed to be a way for a cell in one part of the creature to communicate with cells that are not close by, some sort of highway of intercellular commerce.

The circulation, which is really a series of rivers and canals, arose to answer these needs. Like any system of intricate waterways, sometimes the banks break open and the stream leaks into the surroundings. Our bodies need a way first of plugging the leak and then repairing the hole so that the banks are as strong as they were before. The coagulation cascade, our blood-clotting mechanism, does that job. It faces a unique problem in doing so.

The problem is that blood is a liquid. Like everything inside us, it is based on water and is itself mostly water. The blood cells float along in the stream, and all the other components are dissolved in it. When there is a break in a vessel, whether punctured or completely severed, there is nothing to stop everything inside from rushing out. Immediately after such an accident, this is what happens. The coagulation system must act quickly, which means the components of that system need to be available all the time, ready at hand for any emergency. In essence, the blood must have a way of quickly converting the liquid blood to a solid.

You see in front of you a mass of fibers. Blood cells are trapped in the fibers, and the combination has resulted in a large, solid patch that has stopped further blood from escaping the vessels after your son fell from the tree. It happened fast, because it was only a short time ago that he hurt himself. Where did all those fibers come from? The answer is that they came from the blood itself, which carries with it the building blocks for the fiber meshwork, a substance called fibrinogen.

The fibrinogen remains in liquid form until needed and then, by means of a series of chemical reactions, quickly assembles into a solid. You have probably seen another example of a liquid turning quickly to a solid when acted upon by something else—epoxy glue. In the case of the glue, the two components are kept separate from each other; when they mix, the resin solidifies.

The blood contains the fibrinogen building blocks to make those fibers all around you, which are called fibrin. When the appropriate signal triggers the fibrinogen, the building blocks rapidly come together. Think of the blood as being full of disconnected individual units like interlocking blocks. When the blocks are all in a sack—as when the blood is fluid—you can store the toys under your son's bed; when they are snapped together, especially when they crosslink to each other, the sturdy construction can reach to the ceiling.

If you were to design a blood coagulation system from scratch, ideally, the act of breaking a blood vessel would itself be the signal for the clot to begin forming. That way you would not need an intermediate step of first detecting the break and then mobilizing the response. In fact, this is how the body does it.

On your first trip inside a blood vessel, back in chapter 1, when you visited the infected finger, you took time to look closely at the cells lining the walls. Since then you have been inside so many blood vessels you have stopped noticing them. They appear so ordinary. After all, they have a job as boring as wallpaper, because all they do is line the walls. You are not alone in dismissing their importance; for quite a long time medical researchers did the same thing.

That was a mistake. These lining cells, called endothelial cells, have a crucial job. They are at the nexus point of the immune, inflammatory, and blood-clotting systems. They also are key actors in regulating which blood vessels open and which ones constrict. They are key gatekeepers of the cellular irrigation system, deciding which channels get more blood and which ones get less, according to the body's need at the moment. So you had best go back inside a blood vessel for a moment and look more closely at them.

When you do that and shine your light down the long corridor inside a nearby vessel, you see ranks of flat, cobblestone-like cells. They look like fried eggs in a pan. Crack three eggs into a hot frying pan, and the whites will run over until they touch a neighbor, sealing themselves to the next egg. The bump in the middle of the cell, the yolk in this analogy, is the nucleus of the cell, its nerve center. The perimeter of the cell, like that of the fried egg, is quite thin.

On a couple of your earlier expeditions you saw when there was inflammation in the region, the edges of these cells pulled apart, letting other cells and various blood components out. But most of the time, the small blood vessels are sealed up quite tightly. This is because they are hiding something from the blood; they are concealing the surface that lies beneath the endothelial cells. Even when the small vessels get leaky, when the edges of their endothelial cells pull apart a little, the cells still mostly shield from the bloodstream what lies under them. It is essential that they do this, because what lies below is a powerful trigger for the clot-forming coagulation cascade.

We call blood clotting a cascade because that is what it is—a linked series of events, each of which is set off by something farther up the chain reaction and which, in turn, activates a subsequent step farther down the string of events. At each step the overall effect is amplified to produce more clot.

There are several ways this cascade can get going, but the most powerful trigger is exposure of the surface beneath the endothelial layer to blood platelets. These were those tiny bits of cellular dust you saw budding off larger mother cells when you were in the blood cell factory of the bone marrow. The platelets are miniscule in comparison to complete cells, but they circulate everywhere the blood cells go.

When a platelet spots an exposed bit of tissue beneath an endothelial cell, it immediately attaches to it. Next, it dumps substances that it has stored inside, ready for just such an event. These substances activate other platelets nearby, causing them to do the same thing—more amplification. The platelets also flatten themselves out and stick to both each other and to the exposed surface. In this way they very rapidly grow into a gigantic ball of platelets, forming what we call a platelet plug.

The platelet plug is just the beginning. The surfaces of these newly activated platelets, in tandem with the substances they released into their surroundings, are the signal to the fluid fibrinogen in the blood to transform into the solid fibrin, the strands of a clot. They are like the activator in the epoxy glue package. The reaction in epoxy glue is simple; in contrast, blood coagulation is complicated because there are many steps in the cascade. Only the very last step takes the building blocks of the fibrinogen and links them all together into the solid structure of the clot.

There are other ways for clots to form besides exposing the surface beneath the vessel's lining cells. This is because there are other ways to activate platelets besides exposure of the underside of the endothelial carpet. Some of those inflammatory substances you have been seeing throughout this book—in the infected finger, the sore ear, and around the burst appendix—can activate platelets, which is why we often see some blood clots around inflamed regions of the body. The surface of the endothelial cell lining that faces the bloodstream can, in some circumstances, trigger the cascade on its own.

The coagulation system is a marvelous machine. But the cascade, once activated, poses an immediate problem—how is the body to control this genie once it is out of the bottle? After all, the bloodstream has the equivalent of an infinite number of blocks. What is to prevent the clot from getting bigger and bigger, until every drop of blood inside us is part of an immense clot? That would be a disaster.

Fortunately for us, nature has designed a way out of this conundrum. The instant the coagulation system is activated, the body also turns on an opposing system that blocks the cascade. It even trots out substances that begin to dissolve the very fibrin strands the coagulation cascade is constructing, chopping them into harmless little bits. At first glance, it seems like another situation in which the body uses one crew to dig holes while simultaneously employing another to fill them up as fast as they are dug.

The key to understanding this entire process is to consider the need for balance. In an ideal system, breaks in the blood vessel wall would activate the clotting cascade, forming a patch. But you would not want that patch to be any bigger than necessary, so around its edges you would want to erect a safety zone, a kind of barrier perimeter like a construction fence that separates the injured from the uninjured areas. Inside the barrier, let clotting move along; outside it, shut it off. In effect, this is what the body does. The very nature of the clotting cascade, with its many interconnected steps, provides multiple opportunities to modulate the reaction, fine-tuning so it is just right. All must be in proper balance. Finally, when the job of the clot is done and the hole repaired, it makes good sense to have a method to dismantle the clot and haul it away for disposal. This balance of blood clotting and unclotting is essential to keeping us healthy.

Now that you have renewed respect for what those dull-appearing endothelial cells lining the blood vessels do, it is time to go back out to the broken ends of the bones and investigate what else there is to see. At this point, however, that is not much. The spaces between and around the bone ends are filled with a very large clot. The ends of the bones do not match up, although the orthopedist will soon fix that. What you are looking at is the body's immediate effort at damage control. Healing has not started yet, so to see that drama you will need to come back later. Besides, the orthopedist is ready to go to work, so you leave the scene for now.

After you son wakes up from the effects of the sedatives, the two of you go home. He has a new cast on his arm, as well as some oral pain pills to help him get through the next day or so, because his arm will continue to hurt for a while.

That cast is important for proper healing. It is absolutely crucial for the ends of the broken bones to align and for the ends to remain immobile. The cast accomplishes this, but the orthopedist tells you to watch it very closely. A broken arm always swells, and a cast that goes on when the arm is swollen may be too loose when the swelling goes down—loose enough to let the bone edges move around. Another problem is that the cast can become too tight because of continued swelling and cut off the circulation beyond it. Depending on the individual circumstances, the orthopedist will, on occasion, put on a temporary splint that is sturdy enough to keep the bone edges in the proper place for a day but will stretch a little if there is more swelling. He can then replace that with a more solid cast a day or two later when the swelling has gone down.

In a few days your son's pain is gone. Two weeks later, his arm feels fine, although he complains of some itching under the cast; as you learned last chapter, itching can accompany healing, and the cast can irritate the skin enough to cause itching, too. The last time you visited his arm, all you saw was a mass of clot and some sharp, ragged bone edges. It is time to return and see how things are progressing with his healing several weeks into the process.

When you arrive back at the fracture site, you encounter a cellular building project of immense proportions. You have seen tissue repair before, such as in the finger and the ear, but nothing on this scale. The huge blood clot that obscured your passage before has been riddled full of holes, although remnants remain here and there. Now you can see that, although the bone ends were broken, the membrane covering them, the periosteum, stayed intact. It is draped over and around the broken ends like a tarpaulin covering a construction site. You duck under it to see what is happening.

The first thing you see is that the sharp edges of the broken bone have been smoothed a little. The gap between them has been bridged by a connection of new material called woven bone. Resident bone cells, cells that already lived there and did not need to come from anywhere, made this stuff. Recall when you explored his unbroken arm, you saw an array of apparently quiescent cells, dozing in place until called upon to do something. These cells are now wide awake and busy laying down the scaffolding of new bone. These cells make it possible for bone, unlike some other tissues, to reconstitute itself completely as it was before. What awakened the bone cells were what we call growth factors, and a principal source of these was the huge mass of blood platelets that arrived in the first moments after the injury to begin forming the clot.

The platelets have a short-term and a long-term job. Initially they are part of the damage-control team, but they also are central to healing the injury. Mixed in with the other substances, they dump out powerful growth factors when they first arrive. You cannot see any effect from it immediately, but these substances kick the reparative bone cells into action. Now, a few weeks later, you can see the results. After the framework is in place, the bone cells quickly go to work stiffening it with those hard calcium and phosphate salts, turning it into solid bone. They look like beavers busily repairing a break in their dam to make it just as it was before. Most of this fresh bone is put right beneath the periosteum, re-creating the smooth, hard surface you recall from normal bone, but the inner marrow cavity is also being cleaned and restored.

The growth factors from platelets are a prime stimulus for this rebuilding, but the project has help from other substances released by those familiar cells you have seen at other sites of inflammation, particularly macrophages. The macrophages, as the main tissue cleanup crew, have a huge job following a fracture like this, because they are charged with breaking down the mess into manageable pieces and disposing of them.

In the places where the macrophages have completed their chores, you can see the other repair cells you remember from the infected finger, the fibroblasts. These cells fill in the spaces where the previous cellular residents were too injured by the forces of the breaking bone to go on, so they were marked for demolition by elements of the inflammatory system and carted away by the macrophages. Fibroblasts, which respond to the same menu of growth factors, then reproduce themselves and fill in the holes.

In spite of how well the healing of your son's arm is progressing, it is clear to you that this bone is far from ready to resume its normal function. Before that can happen, the previously broken ends need to be joined together by the hard stuff that gives a bone its strength. The initial, temporary, woven bone is not strong enough to do the job. It will take the bone cells another week or so to complete their task of mineralizing it.

The place where you are now, inside a healing fracture, is called a callous. If you look at it on an x-ray, you can see it as a bump around the edges of where the break was. When the bone is completely healed and hard as before, you usually can still see evidence of a callous, but the bone in it is now as strong and hard as it was before the injury. This is why an x-ray taken even years later of that spot often shows that a fracture was there, just as a major cut on our arm will show a healed scar afterward.

Healing in a bone such as the arm is unique in an interesting way; it is only through ongoing use of the bone later—some weeks after the cast comes off in this case—that the healing process can finish. When the bone is solid, the orthopedist will cut the cast off, and your son will be free to resume his tree climbing. The callous, however, will continue to remodel itself in accordance with the forces of physical stresses it senses. Those cells that break down bone will do their jobs, clearing away some parts of the repair that subsequent use shows were not done in the best way, after which the bone-constructing cells will come back and rebuild. This is why use of an arm or a leg after an injury is important—steady, progressive, normal use, guided by physical therapy for a large break, is key to proper healing. The bone construction crew needs guidance in getting the job done right.

How a broken bone heals is a good prototype for many sorts of injuries. A muscle tear in the leg or a large bruise are other examples. In both these situations, blood spilled into the tissues initially clots then serves to jump-start the cellular healing process. What you saw around your son's broken arm was a specific example of general events that occur throughout the body.

· 9 ·

What Cancer Can Teach Us
about Healing

*H*ealing is intimately bound up in the phenomenon of growth. When tissue is injured, there is inevitable destruction of at least a few body cells, and these cells need to be replaced. As you have seen, especially in the last chapter about broken bones, this process happens when cells respond to messages, called growth factors, which tell them to reproduce themselves. A key related question is why cells do not replicate all the time—what keeps them quiet? Most importantly, what tells them to stop growing when damaged tissue is adequately healed? Do cells get directives not to grow?

The answer to this crucial question is yes: the body controls the prevention of cellular growth as tightly as it controls initiation of it. In fact, the system for damping down cellular reproduction is at least as complicated as the one that switches on cellular growth when healing is needed. For good health the two need to be in balance. Cellular growth—and proper control of it—is essential to our existence.

There is yet another aspect to growth that does not involve healing from injury—normal cellular turnover. You have read in several places how long cells live. Neutrophils, the phagocyte soldiers, often die within hours of their birth. In contrast, memory cells in the immune system can live for many years, possibly as long as we do. We may live as a person, a unique entity, for the biblical "threescore and ten years." Yet in a very real sense that is not the proper way to look at ourselves. We are essentially a large family community of cells. Members of this unique community are continually being born, live out their individual life spans, and then die, even as the community as a whole continues. We only die as individuals when the special entity that is us, this amazing, ongoing collaboration among billions of cells finally quits altogether and all at once.

There are several medical conditions in which the fundamental problem lies in proper regulation of the life span—birth, growth, and death—of the cellular community. Cells cannot be allowed to grow and reproduce without the oversight of the rest of the community, telling them where and how much to grow. If that happens, all the careful, intricate cooperation between body cells goes out the window. Although there are several disorders that fit this description, the one all of us know, and fear, is cancer.

Children do get cancer—not with the frequency adults get it, but it is not uncommon. According to the National Cancer Institute, there were nearly 11,000 new cases among children under age fifteen in 2008. Thankfully, how these children fare has steadily improved over the past decades. According to the same source, in 1970 less than half the children with cancer survived their illness for five years; in contrast, today three quarters of children are alive after ten years. The most common cancer in children, a form of leukemia, or blood cancer, now has a cure rate of 80 percent. Cancer is a serious and often deadly illness. Yet we can learn an enormous amount about healing from studying cancer. We can also learn a great deal about that cellular community that is ourselves. This chapter shows you how that is so.

No parents want to think about the possibility of their child getting this disease, even in the abstract. In spite of that, learning about cancer is worthwhile, because unlocking its inner secrets may one day yield related secrets of not only how to cure cancer, but how best to encourage, coax, and cajole a child's body to heal during all those times when it seems unable to do so on its own.

The first thing to understand about cancer is that every cancer begins with a single cell. When cells reproduce, they do so by dividing into two cells. These two daughter cells each divide into two more cells, and so on. If this process continues unchecked, all the offspring of this single cell, called a clone, can ultimately reach many billions of cells. How fast that happens depends upon how fast they reproduce. If it happens at all depends upon whether the cell listens to the growth-controlling signals it gets both from other, surrounding cells and from inside the particular cell itself.

Cell growth is the basis not only of healing, but also of our continued ability to stay alive. Since very few cells live as long as we do, our body is continually replacing them. When we experience some kind of injury, such as when your son injured his finger or his arm, this rate of cellular replacement revs up even further in order to repair the injury. When the healing is completed, the cells go back to their usual background rate of reproduction. They do this in response to a different set of signals, which tell them that they can relax and go back to their normal duties, since the injury has been fixed. Cancer is fundamentally a derangement in this system of growth regulation—the clone of cancer cells, all of which have a single ancestor, keeps dividing and dividing.

What causes the original cancer cell to go rogue and ignore all the controlling signals it is supposed to heed? The original cause is a change in the cellular machinery, its DNA (short for deoxyribonucleic acid). DNA is the very stuff of life itself. When it goes bad, the cell is likely to go bad, too.

DNA is what we inherit from our parents. With a few exceptions, all our cells have exactly the same DNA, half of which we get from our mother and half from our father. The DNA exists in the center of the cells as long, coiled chains, with each chain closed aligned with another. This alignment is maintained by the component building blocks of DNA, called bases; a base on one strand pairs with its complementary base on the opposite strand.

Much of our DNA actually does nothing at all in our cells; it is left-over material from our distant genetic past, discarded scraps we no longer use. But scattered throughout our DNA chains are specific regions—called genes—that control particular cell functions by serving as blueprints for the manufacture of all the individual components of the cell. We have two copies of each gene, one from each of our parents. Many of the components the genes encode are the things the cells need to do their specialized work. Examples from your travels include the bone cells that make the hard walls of bone and the cells lining the intestines that manufacture the various tools they need to absorb food.

All of us began as a single cell, when our father's sperm met our mother's egg and the two joined. Sperm and egg cells are the exception to the rule that every cell has a duplicate set of genes—one from each parent. These so-called germ cells only have a single copy of each gene. Through a cellular roll of the dice, each germ cell has a fifty-fifty chance of getting one or the other of a parent's particular gene. Once the sperm and egg join into a single cell, their DNA mingles, restoring the two-copy paradigm.

Every cell contains all the DNA we inherit from our parents, so in theory, any given cell could do any given job—it has the blueprints for doing so. This does not happen. This is because as that original fertilized cell divides into more and more cells, a process called differentiation begins, in which some genes became permanently switched off. This is why a bone cell cannot make antibodies; it has the original blueprints for making them, but it does not know how to implement the plans. Differentiation is an important concept for thinking about cancer, because one of the other things that often happens in cancer is that cancer cells find a way to switch on genes they should not be using and thereby do things they should not be doing.

Every time a cell divides into two new cells, it must duplicate its DNA so that each of the daughter cells has a copy. The paired DNA chains unwind and each member serves as the template for making a new matching chain. The process must replicate the several billion base pairs that make up the genetic code without making any mistakes. In actuality, doing that is virtually impossible, and mistakes do happen during the copying process. Relatively speaking, such mistakes are not rare—around one in a million base pairings. Most times these errors, called mutations, are quickly fixed by the cell, which has its own built-in proofreading mechanism. Sometimes the errors remain and can be passed on to its daughter cells when the cell divides again.

There are other ways DNA can change over time. One of several complicated mechanisms can cause stretches of it to move around when chunks of DNA chains are snipped out and exchanged for other pieces in other places. Certain things, such as ultraviolet light and exposure to various chemicals, can alter the DNA.

Overall it is a good thing DNA can change like this. If it could not, we would have no way to adapt and change. Our bodies' cells would have no way to learn new tricks and respond to new challenges. But it is easy to see how mutations could lead to trouble if they happen in some gene that is vital to a cell's survival—a gene that encodes the cellular machinery to take up and use oxygen, for example. Mutations like that are lethal to the cell, so they do not survive to pass on the change to their daughter cells.

Most mutations are not so serious, and most are quite innocent and cause no harm at all. Some can result in disease, such as when a mutation occurs in the gene that is the blueprint for a key cellular component. For example, a mutation in a blood-clotting protein causes the excessive bleeding of hemophilia. Cancer typically begins with a DNA mutation in one of the genes that regulate cell growth. There are several kinds of these growth-controlling genes.

The healing you saw in your son's broken arm had multiple steps, but one of them was the bone cells awakening and starting to reproduce when they read the signals released by the cells around them, such as the platelets. Imagine a mutation that might happen in the cellular gene that begins this growth phase. What if the mutation allowed the cell to turn itself on spontaneously, without any signal from the outside? That could result in out-of-control cellular replication, ultimately leading to cancer.

Cells also have genes that switch off growth, such as when your son's arm was completely healed and the job was done. What if a mutation happened in one of those genes, the ones that shut off growth? If that happened, the progeny of a cell with the mutation would have no built-in stop sign telling them when to become quiet again, when to go back to sleep. That, too, might ultimately lead to cancer.

There is another possibility. As you have read, the great majority of body cells normally have a life span of days or months. This normal cellular turnover is not simply because the cells wear out, although as you have seen, some kinds of cells, such as phagocytes, expend themselves just doing their job. Many other cells die as part of a preplanned chain of events called programmed cell death. It is important that they do this on schedule. If they did not, all of us would accumulate, as just one example, a lifetime total of a couple of tons of bone marrow and several miles of intestines. Programmed cell death is a process we have only recently begun to understand in any detail, but it is clear that many, even most of the body's cells have a built-in clock that tells them when their time is up. Any mutation in the genes that regulate this cellular doomsday clock would have the potential to make the cell and its offspring immortal. Cancer could easily follow.

Yet another possible mechanism for cancer's appearance is a mutation in the genes that control DNA repair. As you read, mistakes in reading and replicating the DNA template are not that uncommon, which is why nature has a system for editing the new DNA strands and fixing the inevitable typographic errors that happen. If a cell has a faulty repair mechanism, it is at risk for future trouble. This is because some errors would inevitably happen in the genes that control growth and cell death. Some of these mistakes slip by anyway, but if a cell is unable to fix any of them at all, the chances of cancer happening are much higher.

Researchers have found that all four of these kinds of mutations are involved in many cancers: an inappropriate start of cellular reproduction where it is not needed, an inability to turn it off once it has started, failure of a cell to die when it is supposed to, and a defective DNA repair mechanism. The common pathway in all of these mechanisms toward cancer is unrestricted, out-of-control cell growth.

Since cancer arises when DNA malfunctions in one way or another, we should not be surprised that a tendency toward cancer does run in families. After all, close family members have similar DNA, so if one family's version of a particular regulatory gene has less ability than that of another family's to ride herd on all the many growth-controlling genes inside a cell, then members of that family would be expected to have a higher risk for getting cancer. That being said, cancer is still a very complicated process. A person's genetic background plays a role, but it is only one actor among many.

A key concept for understanding cancer is that it is a multistep process. Even before researchers knew anything at all about the fine details of DNA and cellular growth, they had practical evidence that it takes more than one event to cause cancer. For one thing, cancer incidence tends to increase with age, which suggested that our bodies had to encounter a string of events as we lived our lives before cancer appeared.

Once scientists had identified many of these growth-promoting and growth-inhibiting genes, they found a demonstration at the cellular level of the same thing—cancer does not happen all at once, but in stages. They analyzed cancer cells for evidence of malfunction in these genes and found that most cancers had multiple defects. Simply altering one growth-promoting gene was not enough. Likewise, it was not sufficient to have a failure in a single growth-suppressing gene. Combined defects in several of these growth-control systems were needed.

A common-sense interpretation of all these esoteric observations is that nature has not put all of her eggs in a single basket. Rather, she has provided our bodies with a series of defenses against cancer, what a security analyst might call "defense in depth." It is only when the last of the defenses has been breached by a succession of attacks that a cell transforms into a cancer cell.

There are many things that have been associated with cancer. Some of these associations are so clear that we can say they cause the cancer. One example is smoking and the most common variety of lung cancer. Others are high-dose radiation, which can cause several types of cancer, and exposure to asbestos fibers, which causes an otherwise rare kind of lung cancer. All of these things do their harm by inducing DNA damage in their target cells. If the exposure is sufficiently high and long, the multiple hits on the system have a progressively higher chance of producing a clone of cancer cells.

Many viruses are known to cause cancer in animals, and it appears that at least some human cancers begin with infections. These viruses all have the ability to insert themselves into the DNA of cells, an action that can alter the function of growth-regulating genes and turn them down the wrong path.

Cancer also can arise in areas of the body where there has been long-standing inflammation and irritation, an observation that shows the relationship between normal healing and cancer's abnormal cellular replication. On your travels around the body you have seen several areas where the cells at the site were participating in a frenzy of new cell production as they worked to replace lost and damaged cells. All the dramas you witnessed had a beginning and an end, when the curtain came down and the audience went home because the show was over. If inflammation continues on and on and on, however, the molecular signals to the local cells continue to whip them along to keep reproducing.

The result of this chronic and intense drive for growth at sites of chronic inflammation is that the cells there go through cycle after cycle of DNA replication. There are persistently high levels of growth factors. There are also large quantities of the molecular weapons inflammatory cells use to attack enemies, but in these chronic situations, the weapons can end up damaging the innocent bystander cells. All of these things make a chronic inflammatory site fertile ground for cellular DNA damage to happen. If a cancer cell randomly appears there, the surrounding rich soup of growth factors can serve to nurture it and encourage it to make others like it. Several kinds of chronic inflammation of the intestinal tract are examples of this process; they carry a high risk of cancer occurring later in the inflamed areas.

The risk of getting cancer affects us all, and does so as long as we live. We can modify the risk by what we do, but we cannot change whatever genetic susceptibility we inherit from our ancestors. Researchers have wondered in the past why we do not all get cancer; put another way, if we lived long enough, would we all get cancer? The increasing incidence of cancer as we age suggests this may be so. Others have asked if cancers actually arise in us now and then—or perhaps frequently—but our bodies are able to contain and destroy them. This idea, that our natural defenses might be able to fight cancer successfully, is fascinating and important to consider if we are to understand cancer and healing. The notion is called immune surveillance, and the idea has been around for decades. The answer to the question of why we do not all get cancer may be that we all do get it, but that some of us are able to eradicate it before it becomes apparent.

The concept of our immune systems—either innate immunity, acquired immunity, or a combination of both—being able to fight cancer is an old one. One reason for the interest is that there have been a few well-documented cases of people recovering from cancer without getting standard treatment or indeed any treatment at all. Such events are rare, occurring perhaps at a rate of one in a hundred thousand instances, but they have happened. You should be very cautious when you hear such claims, especially if the claimant is hawking an untested remedy. But it would be wrong to deny that every once in a while cancer just appears to regress or even disappear on its own.

Another reason for the interest in the possibility of our immune systems helping to fight cancer is that many forms of cancer clearly do provoke an immune response. When we look at the tissues surrounding some kinds of cancer, we can see clear evidence of this. What this implies is that the person's immune system is identifying the cancer tissue as foreign and deserving of destruction. Does this immune reaction do any good—does it ever destroy the cancer successfully? Most importantly, if it does, is there any way to stimulate that response and use it to heal the person?

The main job of the immune system is to identify and hunt down any creature—be it cell, germ, or parasite—that is non-self and thus from the outside. As you have read, nature has developed a complicated yet highly flexible system for teaching the lymphocytes who is friend and who is foe. There are then two principal kinds of lymphocyte soldiers who carry out the attacks: the B-cells make antibodies that attach to enemies and flag them for destruction, and the T-cells instruct and direct the B-cells, as well as deploy certain kinds of special T-cells to attack enemies themselves.

You can think of cancer cells as neither self nor quite non-self. They began as team members but then defected from the team to become something else. In the course of doing that, many cancer cells end up showing on their cell surface unusual proteins, or signposts that mark them as different. These markers have been the focus of many years of research that aims to make a specific vaccine against cancer cells.

Unfortunately, the sort of antibodies you saw work so effectively against germs do not work well against cancer cells. In the laboratory, scientists can induce several kinds of lymphocytes, cells that do not need antibody to work, to attack cancer cells directly and kill them. As of yet, this is as far as the efforts have progressed—promising laboratory research that has not translated into effective cancer treatments.

Because of the promise of the work, however, many scientists persist in the quest to involve the immune system in combating cancer. One reason they continue their quest is that we have some good practical evidence that the immune system must somehow be involved in cancer, even though the overall theory of immune surveillance has not been proven to be true. This evidence is that persons with inherited deficiencies in their immune system have a much higher lifetime risk of getting cancer—about two hundred times higher. This suggests their problems with immunity also give them problems fending off cancer.

All in all, our immune systems do a poor job of helping us fight off and heal from cancer. It is true that immune function declines with age, which may be one reason cancer becomes more common as we get older. In spite of this fact, nearly all people who get cancer have perfectly fine immune systems. Why does their immunity refuse to help? Or does it try to help and fail? The simple answer to these questions is that cancer cells are far more formidable foes than are germs, and they have many strategies to evade destruction.

Now that you know something about cancer, it is time to see how it can affect children and how they can heal from it. This particular story has a happy ending, so no need to worry about how things turn out.

Kyle is three years old. He has always been healthy except for the usual clutch of earaches nearly all toddlers get. Beginning several weeks ago he began to complain that his legs hurt, but otherwise he seemed to his mother to be his normal self. She did notice his legs had quite a few bruises on them. These were mostly on his shins, where one would expect him to bump his legs on the furniture, so she did not pay much further attention to them. A few days afterward his grandmother came to visit and remarked to her daughter how pale Kyle looked. What finally led his mother to bring him to the doctor was finding him in his crib with a nosebleed one morning. As she cleaned him off, she noticed more bruises on his chest and abdomen. That was too much for her, and she brought him in to see what was wrong.

The doctor noticed several things. The boy indeed had more bruises on his skin than you would think to be normal, even for an active three year old. The doctor also noted what Kyle's grandmother had remarked upon: the child was very pale. When she examined the boy she found that his liver, which lies in the upper right portion of the abdomen, just below the ribs, was enlarged and abnormally firm. The doctor also could easily feel his spleen, an organ that is on the upper left side of the abdomen. Normally the spleen is very difficult to feel, because it is nestled high in the abdominal cavity behind the ribcage. Finding it easily with your fingers means that it, too, is enlarged. Finally, some of the lymph nodes in the crease in his groin, what people often term the "glands," felt enlarged.

A simple blood test, called a "complete blood count" because it counts the numbers and relative proportions of the different blood cells, soon confirmed what the doctor suspected—Kyle had a cancer called leukemia. You have made enough journeys through the canals and waterways of the bloodstream to know the usual cells that one finds there. By far the most abundant by a thousand-fold or so are the red blood cells, the pack mules of the circulation that pick up oxygen in the lungs and deliver it all around the body. The white blood cells mostly divide themselves between phagocytes and lymphocytes, both of which cell types you have seen in action as they did their jobs for immunity and inflammation. Sprinkled all around these cells are the fine platelet particles, whose numbers usually are around fifty times the number of white blood cells but still far less than red blood cells.

If you were to look inside Kyle's blood vessels the day he saw the doctor, you would see a very different assortment of cells. The first thing you would notice is that the red blood cells are much reduced; they are only half as numerous as usual. The platelets, too, are much less evident; there are only about a tenth as many as you would normally find. The most dramatic change, however, is the presence of an entirely new kind of cell. It looks sort of like a lymphocyte, one of the B- or T-cells, but it is bigger in comparison to normal lymphocytes.

The unusual cell is called a lymphoblast. The suffix "blast" is shorthand for immature or not completely developed. The lymphoblast is a protolymphocyte that did not develop, or differentiate, to its final form, which would have been a B-cell. Instead, it arrested its developmental pathway at a point before that. This immaturity, along with its explosive and uncontrolled growth, is the mark of cancer.

Kyle has what we call acute lymphoblastic leukemia, a form of blood cancer. Blood cancer can affect any of the blood cell types, but acute lymphoblastic leukemia, or ALL, is the most common one in children. Overall, ALL is the most common cancer of any sort for children.

Since cancer is fundamentally a disorder of cell growth, children with ALL experience out-of-control growth that began with a single abnormal cell of the lineage destined to become a B-cell, an antibody-making cell. This cell escaped all the safeguards you read about earlier in the chapter and began to divide until there were billions of offspring. Along the way, the cells lost their ability to acquire all the normal attributes of mature B-cells, and so all of them are blocked in an arrested state of development. For example, they have no antibody on their surface, because they cannot progress that far in their maturation.

Kyle's symptoms are typical for a child with a new case of ALL, and all of them can be explained by the usual progression of leukemia. The nursery for B-cells is the bone marrow, which is where all those abnormal lymphoblasts were born as well. There are so many of them hatching that the marrow cavity in the middle of the bone stretches due to the pressure inside. There are nerves on the surface of the bones that feel this pressure and transmit it to the brain as pain. This is why his legs hurt.

There are so many lymphoblasts busily reproducing themselves in the bone marrow that they crowd out the normal marrow cells, the ones that make red blood cells, blood phagocytes, and platelets. This is why the blood in his vessels is deficient in all these other types of cells. A deficiency in the phagocytes puts Kyle at some risk for getting infections, since germ fighting is such an important part of the phagocyte's job, but the cancer usually progresses so quickly that is not a problem at this point in a child with ALL.

What often is a problem is the lack of platelets. As you saw in your son's broken arm, those tiny bits of cells are crucial for proper blood clotting. We need them present in sufficient numbers to maintain the normal health and integrity of our small blood vessels, particularly the smallest of these. People lacking enough platelets often experience easy bruising and nosebleeds as Kyle did.

The abnormal lymphoblasts do not confine themselves to just the bloodstream. They also wander out of the circulation, probably because that is what lymphocytes normally do and these immature versions still retain some attributes of normal B-cell function. They go to places where normal lymphocytes go, which are the lymph nodes, the spleen (which is essentially a huge lymph node), and the liver. This is why the examining doctor could feel some enlargement of these in Kyle's body.

The doctor knew as soon as the complete blood count result returned that Kyle had leukemia. But at that point she could not be sure exactly which type he had, since that requires some special tests on the cells. She sent him on to a specialist in these disorders, a pediatric hematologist. Simply because of the statistics, the odds are high that Kyle has ALL, but the hematologist needs to do tests to confirm this, because the best treatments for the different forms of leukemia are not the same. Usually the hematologist needs to take a sample of a child's bone marrow, both to make absolutely sure of the diagnosis and to determine how extensive the leukemia is. Typically nothing needs to be done to the enlarged liver, spleen, and lymph nodes.

These tests take a day or two to finish. When they are done they confirm Kyle has ALL, and he is then ready to start his treatment. In a nutshell, all cancer treatment is aimed at killing cancer cells while sparing normal cells. For many kinds of cancer, this treatment involves surgery to remove as much of the cancer as possible. For some early cancers, just removing it all cures it, because it is still in one spot and has not spread anywhere else in the body.

Most of the time, however, doctors assume that at least a little of the cancer has escaped the surgeon and remains in the person's body. Oftentimes drug treatment, called chemotherapy, is needed to kill these residual cancer cells. Other times radiation therapy, which also kills cancer cells, is the best treatment. Which of these treatments—surgery, chemotherapy, and radiation—works best, and in what combination, depends upon the specific cancer and the individual person.

For ALL, the treatment comes in the form of chemotherapy, because the cancer is not in any single place—it potentially goes everywhere the blood goes and where the immune cells typically congregate. Hematologists have done much research over the years comparing different chemotherapy drugs for ALL. Although they are always looking for drugs that work better or that cause less toxicity than the current standard therapy, for ALL they have a good understanding of what works. This is partly because it is the most common pediatric cancer, so they have had the chance to treat a large number of children.

Since cancer is a disease of disordered growth—of cells growing wildly and without any of the usual restraints—most cancer chemotherapy drugs interfere with cell growth. There are many different categories of these drugs, but they share this common property. For ALL, and many other cancers as well, doctors learned long ago that a combination of different chemotherapy drugs works best. Each of these drugs blocks cell growth using a different mechanism. By combining them together, we can attack the cancer at several different points. If we do not and instead use only one drug at a time, experience has taught us that our chances of curing ALL are much worse than when we use the combination approach.

The standard therapy for a child like Kyle has not changed for the last fifteen years at least. It is a long treatment course, spanning years, and is divided into three phases. The first phase is called induction. It is designed to kill all the cancer cells that are circulating in the blood and those that have come to rest in the various organs. It usually takes a month or two to complete. The way hematologists know that the drugs are working is by monitoring the blood counts in the circulation and by checking the bone marrow for leukemia cells.

Experience has taught us that leukemia cells often make it into the nervous system, and chemotherapy drugs given in the vein do not penetrate very well into the regions around the brain. Thus an important part of induction treatment is to put some of the chemotherapy directly into the fluid that surrounds the brain and spinal cord, called the cerebral spinal fluid. This is done through a needle placed low in the back that goes into the space around the spinal cord. Medicine placed there then circulates all around the spinal cord and the brain.

When we can find no more cancer cells in the blood or the bone marrow, the child is ready for the next phase, called consolidation. Even though we cannot detect any cancer cells in the tests, experience has shown that there are a few lurking somewhere; consolidation is designed to kill these holdouts. Consolidation involves multiple rounds of chemotherapy treatment with breaks in between. It usually lasts six to nine months.

If the tests still show no sign of cancer, then children like Kyle are ready for the last phase of treatment—maintenance. This is less intensive than either of the first two phases and consists of taking smaller doses of chemotherapy drugs on a continuing basis for another couple years. Maintenance is a final safety measure to kill every last one of the cancer cells. Remember that cancer is a disease that begins with a single cell, so killing most of the abnormal cells is not good enough. We need to get them all. If Kyle's tests show no signs of cancer after five years, then the odds are extremely high that he is truly cured. For children like him, we can accomplish this about 80 percent of the time. In our scenario, this is the way matters turned out for Kyle—by the time he is in third grade he is cured of ALL.

As most people know, being treated for cancer with chemotherapy drugs is a long, arduous marathon. This is particularly so for the induction phase and, to some extent, the consolidation phase. This is because chemotherapy drugs are generally quite toxic to the body. They are so toxic that the practical limit to the amount of them we can use is largely determined by pushing the doses as high as possible, to the point where the drug toxicity itself is too dangerous to go higher.

It is the nature of cancer that explains why these drugs are so hard on the body. What all doctors who treat cancer want is a drug that targets only the cancer cells and leaves normal cells alone. In theory this should be possible. Cancer cells often have bizarre derangements from the normal structure and function of the cell type that gave rise to them, and they can have unique markers on their surface that flag them as abnormal. There is ongoing and intense research in which scientists are trying to find ways to design drugs to exploit this fact, but as of yet, this research has not yielded the results we would hope for. Most researchers are confident, though, that we will one day have specific drugs like this.

Until we have something better, virtually all chemotherapy drugs attack cancer by attacking all rapidly growing cells. Since cancer cells are—in comparison to most ordinary body cells—growing rapidly, this means the drugs will preferentially affect the cancer. Unfortunately, there are other cells in the body that also normally grow quite rapidly. These include the cells that line the mouth and the intestinal tract, among others. As you saw when you visited the bone marrow, that particular cell factory is continually churning out red blood cells, phagocytes, and platelets. Because of that, the bone marrow is where many cancer drugs cause the most problems.

Most of the common chemotherapy drugs inhibit normal bone marrow production of blood cells, so a common and even expected complication of treatment is low blood counts. We often have to give children receiving chemotherapy transfusions of both red blood cells and platelets to get them through the induction phase.

The phagocytes present a special problem because they are so important in fighting off infections. For various technical reasons, transfusions of these do not work well. We do have medicines we can give to kick-start the marrow into making more of them, but low counts of these cells is a frequent problem during treatment. Children with very low phagocyte counts are often dangerously susceptible to infections.

These infections generally come from the places in the body you might predict, based on the knowledge you gained during your earlier explorations. Places where lots of bacteria are very close to places where bacteria should not be—where keeping the bacteria at bay is a constant struggle—is where bacteria can gain the upper hand when the phagocyte counts are low. The respiratory tract is one such place. A particular danger zone is the intestinal tract, since the density of bacteria living there is extremely high. When a child's phagocyte count drops, the bacteria can seize their chance and invade.

For this reason we need to watch very closely for signs of infection, particularly fever, anyone receiving chemotherapy whose phagocyte numbers are very low. When that happens we use immediate treatment with powerful, intravenous antibiotics and sometimes reduce the chemotherapy dose to allow the bone marrow to recover—in a sense, to come up for air—and produce more of the essential phagocytes.

Kyle is cured of his leukemia, but his life will never be quite normal again. This is because cancer drugs are a double-edged sword. The same drugs that kill the cancer cells can affect the DNA of normal body cells, causing them to change or mutate. Since mutation of DNA is the first step in cancer, cancer-curing drugs can also be cancer-causing drugs. It is uncommon, but unfortunately it is not rare. For the rest of his life, Kyle will be at risk for a second cancer, one caused by the treatment for his first one. This is why much current research in ALL treatment concerns trying to figure out a way to determine doses of chemotherapy drugs that are sufficient to cure the cancer but have the lowest risk of causing a second cancer years later.

Children heal from cancer a bit differently than they heal from the other problems you have seen. You are familiar now with how the immune and inflammatory systems range throughout the body, working in much the same way wherever they go. The local circumstances of a particular body part matter, as you have also seen, but the similarities of healing dwarf the differences.

In contrast, the body is helpless against cancer nearly all of the time. After surgery, radiation, and chemotherapy have done their job as best they can, the body's cellular cleanup crew can move in and heal the battlefield, cart away all the dead cancer cells, and recycle their component parts, as it does for all other spent cells. But in spite of all the research, we have not yet discovered a consistent way of awakening the body to the danger, activating its natural defenses, and taking care of the cancer on its own. I do think that is coming in the future, perhaps the near future. The rare instances of apparently spontaneous cures entice us with the possibilities, but we are not there yet.

· 10 ·

How Can We Help a Child Heal?

$\mathcal{B}$y now you have seen, and even experienced to some extent, the wide range of events taking place throughout a child's body as it heals. One goal of all your expeditions was to make those things vividly real to you; parents can see what is happening to their sick children on the outside, but can only guess at what is happening on the inside. Another goal was to show you how the cellular and molecular drama explains the symptoms your child has, how he feels. A final goal was to show you how all those places—ears, lungs, intestines, and bones—look afterward. These are good things for parents to know. But what most parents really want to know is what they can do to improve things, to speed healing along. This chapter concerns what we know about ways you can do that.

The first category of healing aids to consider are the straightforward, concrete ones—things you can do to the sick or injured body part itself. As you saw on your visits to both the injured finger and sore ear, in both of these places the cells must first clean up a fairly large mess before much serious healing can happen. This is true for any site in the body where collections of pus—that mixture of phagocytes, germs, and cellular debris—occur. Although many of the germs are dead, the pus typically contains some living bacteria, as well as hefty amounts of all those substances released by phagocytes and macrophages that serve to fuel the inflammatory fire. Healing cannot really start until these things are cleared away, and often we can help the body accomplish this.

Soaking a small abscess in warm water, as you did for your son's finger, is one simple way to help remove the pus. For larger abscesses, physicians often lance them open to drain them out, although this is not something you should try at home. One reason to leave it to the doctor is that, incorrectly done, you can make things worse by introducing bacteria into the bloodstream. Another reason is that lancing an abscess hurts; the doctor can use medications to numb the area.

Abscesses deep inside the body often require a more involved surgical procedure to remove the pus. For small abscesses, such as the one you saw in the finger, the body would eventually have taken care of matters by itself without any help. For larger abscesses, however, draining them is often necessary to get them to heal completely. Physicians have known this for thousands of years. They learned it from watching nature at work, seeing how things healed faster after an abscess ruptured and drained spontaneously.

Once an abscess opens, either on its own or with our help, it is important to keep the area clean and dry. This keeps fresh germs from getting inside and causing mischief. A thin film of antibiotic ointment (not a large glop of it) helps to keep the area germ free and to protect the healing cells underneath.

Nature protects a superficial wound with her own bandage—the familiar scab. It is a crust made up of a mature blood clot and dried cellular debris that covers the place where the skin was broken. Until the area is completely healed, it is best to leave a scab alone and open to the air. But since the healing area often itches, sometimes it is difficult for a child not to pick at a scab. When that happens, bleeding often starts again. The reason a picked scab—especially a large one—can bleed so exuberantly is because, as you have seen, part of cellular healing is bringing a good blood supply to the site, in the form of a maze of fresh capillary vessels. When you rip off the roof of the cellular construction site, those new tiny spots tend to bleed.

The principle of removing cellular debris also applies to inflammation elsewhere, even if there are no infecting germs present. An example of this is the lung after an asthma attack. The breathing treatments your son got during his asthma episode helped open up his airways to let air in and out, and he also got several other medications to help diminish the inflammation around his airways and reduce the mucous production. That halted the process, but there was still a substantial amount of mucus and cellular debris clogging his breathing tubes that had already built up. Getting that stuff up and out of his breathing tubes speeds healing.

The way to clear it out is to cough. This is an important principle for a wide variety of lung problems besides asthma, particularly pneumonia. Any inflammatory process that produces excess mucus ultimately relies on the person coughing to get the stuff out of the lungs. The asthmatic is troubled mostly by mucus; in the case of pneumonia, the mucus often is more like pus, laden with phagocytes and germs. In those circumstances, coughing it out is akin to draining an abscess, and it has the same beneficial effect.

Physicians have known for a very long time that it is often when a patient with pneumonia is improving overall—less fever, better appetite, less trouble breathing—that coughing up mucus is more prominent. This is because, as they recover, the healing airways are shoveling the mucus up to the larger breathing tubes so the child can cough it out. So a day or so of a worsening cough is often a sign of healing.

Cough is also an important way to expand the lungs fully after a prolonged period of not using them very much, such as when a child lies for several days in a hospital bed after major surgery, not getting any exercise that would normally make her use her lungs to their fullest extent. This is one reason why a standard part of therapy after surgery is to encourage the patient to take deep breaths and cough. Besides these effects of temporary disuse on the lung, the anesthetics given during surgery actually slow down the lung's normal debris-removal system, the cilia, and mucus tends to build up as a result. Coughing helps get everything moving again.

As you read in chapter 7, relieving some kinds of symptoms speeds healing, while relieving other symptoms may have the opposite effect. Pain, especially moderate to severe pain—such as that which follows broken bones or major surgery—causes activation of the body's emergency stress response system. These are the "fight or flight" hormones that are initially useful for our response to injury, because they help our systems cope with big, important issues like shock and blood loss. These same hormones, however, can subsequently interfere with tissue healing by inhibiting the ability of the cellular actors at injury sites to play their proper roles. Relieving pain helps healing in this way. Relieving itching helps healing by keeping us from repeatedly reinjuring the spot by scratching it, interrupting the itch-scratch cycle.

It is unclear if treating fever helps, hurts, or has no effect on healing. If blocking fever does interfere with healing just a little, most doctors believe the trade-off to be a good one, because fever can make a child miserable. You could easily argue that relieving that kind of discomfort should help overall, just as relieving pain does. On the other hand, fever does not bother some children much. If your child is like this, realize it is reasonable not to treat the fever just because it is there. Nature is wise, and fever is clearly part of your child's natural response to illness.

There are several things we can do to speed the healing of injuries. You visited a broken bone, a more severe example, but most children's injuries are more minor than that. A sprain, for example, is an injury that stretches and sometimes tears the ligaments—the tough, fibrous bands of tissue that surround, support, and protect joints. Muscle injury often comes from a blow directly to the muscle or by stretching it too far, pulling some of the fibers apart.

The standard treatment for these kinds of injuries is rest, ice, compression, and elevation. This scheme is often abbreviated with the acronym RICE. You now know enough about what goes on inside injured tissues to understand how these four things aid healing.

The first component, rest, is to prevent continuing the injury process by using the arm or leg unnecessarily while it is trying to heal. The fracture you saw was an extreme case; if you do not immobilize the bone ends, they will never heal properly. The cast is a way of resting the area by physically preventing its use. Lesser injuries—such as stretched and bruised ligaments over a twisted ankle or a finger bent backward—benefit from the same thing. When we place a sprained ankle in a splint or wrap it with supportive tape, we are giving it a rest and improving its ability to heal rapidly.

Inflammation produces heat, and heat prolongs inflammation. Most of us know this well, which is why putting an ice cube on a fat lip reduces the swelling. When a baseball pitcher ices his elbow, he is heading off the inflammation that long innings of pitching often brings on. An astute reader might well ask, though, if suppressing inflammation with ice is a good thing. After all, a major theme of this book has been that inflammation is a natural process that aids healing. The best answer to this argument is that standard amounts of cold treatment, such as with cold compresses and ice packs, do not shut off inflammation completely; there will always be enough there sufficient for the body's needs. The effect of mild to moderate cooling is to take the edge off, inhibiting enough of the inflammatory reaction to reduce pain and swelling, but still allowing enough to promote healing.

The last two components of the acronym, compression and elevation, go together. An elastic bandage wrapped around an injured arm or leg, for example, coupled with keeping the afflicted part higher than the heart so the circulation tends to run downhill, reduces the swelling already present and heads off further swelling to come. That swelling, of course, is the result of the inflammatory process you know so well.

After a day or two, when RICE has done its work, a sore arm or leg heals faster if we progressively use the injured area in a controlled way, taking care not to injure it again through overuse. Avoiding reinjury is where the symptom of pain can be helpful; if it hurts too much when we start using it again, we are probably going too fast or pushing it too hard. This can be a tricky balance, so after a significant twist or sprain, it is useful to get specific advice on how to proceed from your child's doctor or a physical therapist. There are several good reasons for this approach.

As you saw in the finger, healing often involves scar formation by those busy fibroblasts, which can cause a drawing together, or contraction, of the tissues. This is especially true for larger injuries. For a skin injury, such as a large cut, that is what we want to happen. Even though the scar may be a little unsightly, it is nature's way of sealing up the skin properly. However, that sort of scar formation can be a problem for a deeper injury, such as an injury around a joint or in a major muscle. Rehabilitation—proper physical therapy—is intended to keep the area limber during the later phases of the healing process to ensure this does not happen. Once a deep, unwanted tissue contraction has happened, it is difficult to correct, so it is better to prevent it from happening in the first place.

For a broken bone, proper rehabilitation serves an additional purpose. As you saw, bone is an unusual tissue. If you just put a child with a broken bone to bed, the ends will knit together if they are touching one another. But the bone will not resume its normal state—its previous architecture—unless you use it as it was intended. Progressive use of a broken limb needs to be done carefully so that it is not done too soon, before the previous break is sufficiently solid to tolerate the exercise and weight, but it should not be done too late, either. Parents need guidance about how to do this correctly. The final stages of bone remodeling, of finishing the job of mending it completely, do not happen until a child uses that bone again to do its job.

Draining pus, coughing up residual phlegm and mucus, relieving pain, and rehabilitating injuries are all specific measures for aiding healing. What about more general measures, things like getting enough rest for the body, eating well, and having a positive attitude? These are all platitudes our parents and grandparents have passed on to us, perhaps in a nagging way: "Of course you feel rotten—you don't eat right and you don't get enough sleep." Is there anything to these admonitions? Just what do we know about the role of nutrition in healing? Does a positive mental outlook help healing, and a negative, depressed way of looking at the world interfere with it? And what about alternative therapies, those outside the medical mainstream? What do we know about their effects on healing?

Healing is hard work for the body, and hard work requires energy. We can get energy from only two places: we can reach into our body's larder where it is stored, or we can take in new energy through what we eat. Both are important for healing. It is true that most of what we know about this issue comes from studying more extreme examples of illness and injury than those we have considered in this book. Even so, we have reason to think the principles that apply to more serious situations also are relevant to everyday examples of how children heal.

We know quite a lot about the body's use of energy immediately after sickness starts or injury occurs. Illness brings with it a need for more energy; the immune and inflammatory events represent a large uptick in energy use because all those cells need fuel on which to run. The body also needs new cellular recruits for the battle, and most of these new cells need to be made. The sudden, massive increase in output of the cell factories in the bone marrow is evidence of this phenomenon.

A sick child's body also burns energy in other ways. Newly released stress hormones raise what we call the basal metabolic rate, the body's background energy consumption. It is similar to your car's engine when it is idling. If you increase the idle setting, you increase the amount of gas your car burns. Fever, which accompanies many illnesses, brings its own demands for increased energy. As a rough rule of thumb, each degree of fever causes a 10 percent increase in the body's baseline calorie needs.

In the early phases of acute illness, a child takes both the additional needed energy and the building blocks for all these new cells from within herself. We all have reserve supplies of these materials, and the body is very good at recycling components of old cells to make new ones. This is why we can still keep our blood sugar, the principal fuel, in a good range even if we do not eat for many hours: our liver releases a steady trickle in amounts sufficient to keep the level normal. This is important because, besides oxygen, our body's cells do not do well when deprived of fuel. This is particularly so for the heart and the brain: both need around-the-clock feeding.

Knowing that serious illness or injury puts a drain on the body's reserve energy supplies, it seems logical that it would be a good thing if we could short-circuit this reflex by providing extra calories when a child is sick. This would spare the need for the child's body to go to its supply pantry, plus provide an added energy boost for the child. It is a sensible idea, but unfortunately it does not quite work that way.

The stress hormones direct the early response to serious illness or injury, the mobilization of energy from the body's storehouse. These hormones direct the body to use its reserves, even if it means breaking down tissues to scavenge the supplies. For good measure, these hormones also inhibit the ability of the intestine to absorb nutrients, so the digestive system ignores what food is there. The hormones even suppress the appetite, which is the main reason sick children do not feel like eating much. All these things mean that giving extra calories (or extra protein or any other nutrients) in the initial phase does not change how the body responds to stress.

Even though feeding your child extra calories in the acute stage of illness does not speed healing, there is an important dietary intervention parents can do that is important—ensuring your child gets sufficient fluid. As a group, small children need more fluid each day relative to their body mass than older children and adults do. This is because their relative surface area is higher, and they radiate more heat and moisture to the outside world. Fluid is different from calories and other nutrients, because the body cannot go to some internal storehouse and produce it, as it can with energy. To get fluid, the body will rob some areas to supply others, particularly keeping the bloodstream as full as possible. When it does that, net fluid loss results—dehydration.

Avoiding dehydration is important for healing because, in spite of all the cells and proteins in it, the blood is primarily water. Indeed, the entire body is mostly water—about 60 percent. Those cellular processes you saw at work around healing areas do best when there is good circulation, which means adequate amounts of water. This is especially so in children, who are much more prone than adults to suffer the adverse effects of dehydration. Thus, keeping your child well hydrated when she is sick is a simple but important measure you can take to promote healing.

Doctors use a formula to calculate how much fluid a child needs. It is an easy formula to master, and it provides a good guide for parents. It is based upon body weight, which doctors express in kilograms, but one can easily convert it to a useful rough guide using pounds. Relatively speaking, the smaller the child, the larger the amount of fluid he needs, adjusted for body weight.

A common version of the formula divides children into three categories: less than twenty-five pounds, twenty-five to fifty pounds, and over fifty pounds. The first group needs about a half teaspoon of fluid each hour for each pound of body weight. This means a ten-pound child needs five teaspoons an hour, which is a little more than two thirds of an ounce, or roughly about two ounces every three hours. A twenty-pound child needs twice that—about four ounces every three hours.

The second group of children, those weighing twenty-five to fifty pounds, need about four to six ounces every three hours, and the biggest children about six to eight ounces every three hours. A cup of juice is usually about four ounces and a large glass closer to eight ounces. So offering you child something to drink every three to four hours should keep them well hydrated.

These are rough guides and are the most useful for the smallest children, but worth writing down somewhere handy as a rule of thumb when your child is sick. For a child of any age, a good gauge of adequate fluid intake is if the child is urinating normally. If your sick child is wetting her diapers normally, her fluid situation is probably fine; conversely, if your twelve-year-old son with the flu has not been to the bathroom for eight hours, it is a good idea to get him to drink more. Remember to increase the amount of fluid if your child is also losing fluid, such as through vomiting or diarrhea, or if she has fever.

Going beyond the importance of adequate fluids, researchers have known for decades that nutrition is closely connected to healing. For example, people who are malnourished have demonstrable reductions in their immunity. The practical evidence for this is that poorly nourished people, especially children, get a lot more infections than their well-fed peers. Further, once they get these infections, malnourished people have much more difficulty fighting them off because their immune and inflammatory mechanisms are sluggish. Researchers can isolate some of the immune cells from the blood—lymphocytes, phagocytes, and macrophages—and challenge them in the laboratory to do their job. Malnourished people show poor function of many of these cells, indicating that poor nutrition affects many aspects of immunity.

General tissue healing, such as after an injury or surgery, is also markedly affected by the person's nutritional state. Malnourished people do not heal well. A good example of this is found in several kinds of chronic intestinal disorders that cause malabsorption of food. Surgeons found long ago that people with those problems, if they need an operation, are at great risk for poor healing and other complications, unless they first get their nutritional status improved.

This information is all interesting, but it is not unexpected. After all, healing is hard work for the body and takes energy and resources from the body; therefore, we would predict problems with healing if a person's nutritional storehouse was poorly stocked for emergencies. But few children are malnourished, so their reserves are normal. Besides, as you read, because of the stress response, extra food does not help healing in the initial stages of significant illness or injury. But what about later? Can extra nutrition for a child who is not otherwise malnourished—who was normal before he got sick—help healing after the acute stages of the illness have passed?

For a child with a very serious illness or injury, such as one that would land him in an intensive care unit, we believe the answer is yes—extra nutrition helps healing. The reason is not that super-calories speed healing; instead, it is that the daily nutritional needs of a very sick child in the healing phase are much higher than normal. We have ways of estimating what those extra needs are and strive to provide them. We know if we do not, healing can be delayed.

Thankfully, most sick or injured children are not critically or even seriously ill. They just have problems like infected fingers, earaches, or simple broken bones. They were perfectly well grown and healthy before they got sick. What about them? Does loading in some extra nutrition when they are sick or injured help them heal?

The answer to that practical question is no—extra calories do not help. Still, many parents notice that as a child recovers from illness and his appetite returns, he will often be hungrier than usual for a time. If he has been sick for more than a day or so, you may notice that he has lost a little weight. No doubt this extra appetite when he starts to recover is nature telling him to restock his body's larder.

It is useful to think of nutrition in another way besides calories. Food is not merely food. For children—and adults, too—food also means comfort. Often food means love. This connection between nutrition and emotion is a good way to begin a consideration of the enormous and fascinating body of research connecting mental state with healing.

There is no question that the brain and the body are directly connected to each other. After all, our heads sit squarely atop our shoulders, and anatomists can draw the physical links in great detail. In spite of this obvious physical truth, both philosophers and ordinary people have been vexed for millennia over what is often termed the "mind-body problem." Does the mind, our consciousness of ourselves as individuals, exist as a thing separate from our brains, the physical place where our consciousness lives? Or does our consciousness consist of nothing more than the sum of all our brain cells?

Philosophers being philosophers, there is no agreement among them on this question. What is called dualism, the notion that mind and body are discrete and separate entities, has long had champions in Western philosophical tradition. It is easy to see the appeal of preserving a mystical separation between our awareness and the organ than facilitates that awareness—our brains. The nerve cells in our brains communicate with one another by exchanging chemical messages with one another. It is a sobering thought to regard our consciousness as consisting simply of the summation of billions of such messages, which together somehow allow awareness to me as I write this and to you as you read it.

There remain some philosopher-dualists, but these days it is very hard to find a neuroscientist, or a brain researcher, who does not think that eventually with enough research we will understand how all those microscopic bursts of chemicals in the brain of a person studying the brain allows her to be conscious of analyzing her own consciousness.

Using our alert and focused brain we carry out conscious acts. That same brain also hums along in the background, beneath the level of our awareness, doing an enormous number of unconscious activities. It keeps our heart beating and tells our intestines to move food along without us having to think about it. Yet it quickly links these so-called autonomic functions to consciousness when fear or excitement makes our heart rate double or gives us nausea. We have obvious evidence such as that of the many direct connections between the mental construct of ourselves and the actual reality of our bodies.

Is there any evidence that mental state—what is happening in our brains—can affect healing? In fact, there is an enormous amount of information that suggests this is so. The data range widely in quality, from well-conducted, scientific studies (the minority) to testimonial anecdotes (perhaps the majority), some of which strain credulity. The field is so broad we can consider here only a small sampling of it, focusing on research that applies to what you in your microscopic journeys have seen happening in healing children.

The first question to consider is if events in the brain can interfere with healing. You already have a partial answer to that question. Pain is something perceived and interpreted by the brain, and constant pain can delay healing by activating the stress hormone response. Not surprisingly, other forms of stress can do the same thing. In a sense, it is a way of demonstrating something we all know: not all pain is physical, and mental anguish can have the same effect.

An easily studied form of healing is that of superficial skin wounds. It is a useful model because it can be standardized among individual subjects. In both humans and experimental animals, skin wounds take longer to heal when the individual is subjected to psychic stress. Examples of the sorts of stresses researchers have studied include students around examination time, couples experiencing marital stress, and general anxiety around the time of major surgery.

Depression is another example of a mental state that research strongly suggests can affect healing. A variety of studies indicates that depressed people do not recover as quickly from either simple, superficial wounds or from the more extensive injury of major surgery, as compared with people who are not depressed. These research studies strongly suggest that what goes on in the mind can have profound effects on how the body heals.

If it is true that untoward mental events can interfere with healing, what about the reverse? Can a highly positive outlook speed healing? Is there any hard evidence for the old idea that there is healing power in positive thinking? Can thinking good thoughts make us get better faster? And what about medications that treat anxiety and depression? If all brain activities derive from the exchange of chemical messages between nerve cells, we would expect depressive and anxious thoughts to be governed by these chemical events. Although the appropriate role for using antidepressant drugs, medications that alter these chemical exchanges, is controversial—many think they are prescribed too liberally—what is not in debate is the fact that we can alter mood with all manner of drugs. Can doing this sort of thing encourage healing, or might it make healing move slower?

We want and need answers to these questions, but it is important to realize this kind of research is difficult to do. The most powerful kind of medical research is the kind in which we take a population of people with a particular condition, divide them into two groups, do some kind of intervention in one group but not the other one, and compare the results. This is called a controlled trial. It works best if the assignment of people to each group is totally random and if neither the investigator nor the patients knows which group they are in until after the trial is over.

Such randomized, controlled trials are the gold standard for medical research. In many situations, however, they are nearly impossible to do. The intervention, such as a surgical procedure, may be impossible to do blindly—the investigator or the patient can easily figure out which group they are in. If the intervention is a drug, the investigator typically blinds the study by giving the "no intervention" group a useless pill, called a placebo. But even that safeguard may be difficult to accomplish in practice if the drug being tested produces some effect, say a funny taste in the mouth, that makes it clear who is in what group. We can reduce this problem by having another investigator, one who does not know which group is which, analyze the data, but it is still a potential problem.

If the intervention is intended to affect the person's mental state, such as relaxation, yoga, exercise, or many other similar activities, blinding the investigator to which person is in which group can be very difficult indeed. Finally, the bias of the investigator—perhaps she really, really wants to show the intervention helps—also easily affects how she measures the results. She is liable to interpret everything in a positive light. In spite of these pitfalls, there is a large body of research about mental health interventions and healing that suggests improving mood, outlook, and overall mental state can speed healing.

If healing is inhibited by stress, it makes sense that relieving stress will remove that inhibition and improve healing. Accordingly, simple relaxation techniques are obvious targets for research and have been extensively investigated over many years. Much of this research has focused on adults undergoing treatment for cancer.

Daily relaxation, even for periods as short as a half hour or so twice each day, does lower blood levels of stress hormones, as well as bring down blood pressure and lower heart rate, two simple physiologic indicators for how active these stress hormones are in the body. Daily meditation, which combines relaxation and a conscious effort to increase self-awareness, can do the same thing. Think of it as a way of emphasizing the mind-body connection. For adults, these improvements clearly have practical outcomes—they aid healing.

Children are not like adults, and many of the structured relaxation and meditation techniques taught to adults do not work for the very young. In spite of that, all parents know there are many ways to calm and soothe their children to relieve their anxiety. Can doing those things help their children heal?

The subject of mind-body interactions in children is sufficiently vast that a specific example is the best way to get a handle on the topic. Asthma is an excellent choice for this. It is common and doctors have long known that although environmental triggers play a huge role in setting it off, the inner psychological state of the child also is important. Asthma is a complex disorder in the way emotional and environmental factors interact with each other, but in spite of that fact asthma is not mysterious and subtle; it causes easily measurable physical effects in a child that correlate to well-known cellular events deep in the lung. You have seen these things happen yourself.

Asthma is a breathing problem, so it makes sense that many of the attempts to influence mind-body interactions in asthma patients center on breathing. The ultimate goal would be to reduce the frequency and severity of airway inflammation, as well as the constriction of the airways. There have been so many studies of this kind with asthma that a highly respected research organization called the Cochrane Collaboration (www. cochrane.org) has been able to do an analysis of what, in sum, all these investigations tell us. Their conclusion is that psychological interventions in asthma do improve symptoms in children as well as adults. The effect is not a strong one, but it is real and can be objectively measured.

There is thus solid but indirect evidence that the brain can somehow influence processes that involve both inflammation and immunity. We have some suggestive direct evidence about how this might happen. Immune cells, such as lymphocytes, have receptors on their surface for several of the chemical messages the brain cells use to talk to one another, the neurotransmitters. This means the connections are normally there for potential conversations between brain cells and those of the immune system.

Clinical depression reduces several cellular measures of immune function. Stress does this, too. A good practical indicator of this is the observation that many people who have occasional cold sores on their lips tend to get them when they are experiencing some sort of emotional stress. Cold sores are caused by a reactivation of a latent herpes virus that many of us have in our nerves, a painful event encouraged by any lapse in our immune function. For many people, that lapse accompanies some form of physical stress, such as another infection, or mental stress.

Wading into the vast amount written about connections between mind and body can be a maddening experience. In the Internet age you can find a confusing welter of claims and counterclaims about what is going on and why. Yet one cannot escape the conclusion that our psyche, our emotions, and our sense of well-being are all tied to healing.

Enough theory—to a parent with a sick child looking for practical advice, it boils down to this: your child's comfort, anxiety level, and general level of irritation most likely affect in some way her ability to heal. The association may not be a strong one, but optimizing these things makes sense. Compared to adults, children are generally happy and optimistic little creatures. On average, children also heal better and faster than adults. Of course, a child's body is fresher and newer than an adult's body, and this fact probably explains much of the reason it heals easier. Yet it seems reasonable to surmise that a child's mostly sunny disposition and good healing capacity are somehow related at the cellular level.

The children in this book have gotten antibiotics for an earache, inhaled medicines for wheezing, undergone an operation for appendicitis, and chemotherapy for leukemia. These are all standard treatments, the stuff of mainstream medicine. As most parents know, there is an entire parallel treatment world, loosely called complementary and alternative medicine, or CAM for short. Estimates are that at least a third of all adults use one or more of the various components of CAM, and presumably many of these are parents who use these remedies on their children as well.

Complementary and alternative medicine is a huge treatment universe, so huge that even regarding it as a single system is unrealistic. It encompasses herbal therapy, acupuncture, massage therapy, homeopathy, relaxation therapy, and much, much more. Even these broad categories contain a myriad of subcategories. Each one of them has its own theories of action, some of which even conflict with each other. But a parent with a sick child—especially a child who has been sick for some time and has not yet healed—generally is not interested in theories; a parent wants to know if any of these things can help.

The effectiveness (or lack thereof) of CAM is a contentious topic, complete with books with incendiary titles arguing both sides of the issue. CAM practitioners are labeled charlatans and quacks; CAM critics are called small-minded and ignorant in their refusal even to consider the possibility that anything outside standard medical paradigms could be helpful.

It is difficult to sort out who is right and who is wrong, especially because many forms of CAM are not really amenable to being investigated by the usual gold standard of randomized, controlled trials. Physical interventions are hard to disguise from the person getting them, although there have been several trials comparing sham acupuncture, done in the theoretically wrong spots, with real acupuncture. Many CAM treatments are not standardized in any way, so it is impossible to choose which way of doing things to compare to standard medical practice.

There is also big money at stake, which naturally ramps up the venom coming from both sides. Some strident CAM opponents cry fraud, and more than a few extreme proponents answer with accusations of monopolistic restraint of trade by physicians afraid of the competition. Can parents take away anything practical from all of this, find anything useful?

Here is how I look at it. There certainly are occasions when, against all predictions from the doctors, people recover and heal from illnesses. When these things happen, nature is teaching us that we do not know as much about her as we think we do. She also may well be reminding us of the links between mind and body, particularly those that connect the brain to the immune and inflammatory systems, the chief mediators of body healing. An inner sense of comfort and well-being reinforces our powers to heal, and anything that promotes it is bound to help.

It does not surprise me that when a patient believes a treatment will work, it often helps. This is often called the "placebo effect," but that term can hang an unnecessarily pejorative construction on what is happening. As you have read, attitude and emotions have demonstrable effects on healing. The effect is not predictably consistent and it is not large, but it is real.

Of course, if parents choose to try one or more aspects of CAM, they should at least be very sure that the treatment does no harm—some CAM modalities are potentially harmful. They also should not replace traditional medical therapies of proven effectiveness with unproven CAM treatments. If those conditions are met, I have no objection at all to parents giving CAM a try. There are many doctors who feel the way I do. Some even use CAM themselves or recommend it to their patients. So it is a mistake not to tell your child's doctor when you are using some aspect of CAM for your child's illness. If doctors are to do their best for children, they need to have all the information.

· 11 ·

When Healing Fails

$\mathcal{C}$hildren are amazingly resilient. Nearly all of the time they heal quite well from whatever illness or injury afflicts them. But sometimes this happy result does not occur. Sometimes healing is incomplete. On rare occasions it does not happen at all. This chapter is about some of the reasons for these unsatisfactory outcomes.

By now you understand that healing is not a mysterious, magical process; it is an intricate, but fairly well understood progression of events. Way back in the first chapter we compared this process to a play. Another useful way to think of it is as a dance, a ballet. After all, the cellular actors are not simply speaking to one another through chemical messages; they are also moving about in an intricately choreographed cellular dance. In the previous chapters you met all the chief cellular actors and dancers in the production, both the heroes and villains. You also saw that the play largely divides itself into three acts.

First come the events that disturb the routine of the body's usual activities, such as invasion by germs or injury. This opening act ends with the body's cellular rapid-response team assembling at the site, where they carry out their initial reconnaissance duties, assess the situation, and mobilize whatever additional resources they need to contain and then reverse the harm. The curtain then opens on the second act, displaying these cellular characters at work as they contain the damage, destroy any unwanted invaders from the outside, and set the stage for the third act. The final act, often the longest of the drama, shows the members of the cellular clean-up and reconstruction crews arriving on the stage and doing their best to restore the site to the way it was before. When they are finished, the curtain comes down on the drama and the audience goes home.

One way healing can fail is because the players do not follow the script. This can happen during any of the three acts, but for children a common reason for not concluding, or even reaching the third act, is persistent inflammation. You could think of this as a failure of the second act's players to leave the stage when they should. Inflammation is a powerful weapon for healing, but it does inflict unavoidable collateral damage on the surrounding tissues. The more extreme the inflammation, the worse the potential damage. Thus, it is important for the body to limit inflammation to where and when it is truly essential. Act two needs to end before the characters in act three can do their job.

A common cause for persistent inflammation is the continued presence of something that provokes the inflammatory system and its frequent coworker, the immune system. One example of this is the persistence of an outpost of enemy microbes, a sanctuary safe from the body's defenses, from which they can conduct a sort of guerrilla war against the body. You have already seen several potential examples of this.

Recall your visit to your son's infected finger in chapter 1. The way that infection got started was through a splinter he picked up while hammering boards together. The splinter breached the primary defense against infection for most of our body, the skin, and carried a vanguard of invading bacteria into the normally sterile microworld of his fingertip. Once there, the bacteria began rapidly to reproduce. In effect, they knew they had only a few hours or so before the cellular defensive soldiers arrived in strength, and they wanted to be ready with as many comrades-in-arms as possible when that happened.

Once the battle in the fingertip between germs and phagocytes truly began, you tilted the balance in favor of your son's defenses by eliminating the microbes's hiding place; you removed the splinter by soaking your son's hand in a bowl of warm water. If that splinter had remained in place, for example, by breaking off and embedding its tip itself deep inside, it would have served as a continuing fortress for the germs, making it much more difficult to heal his finger.

On your trips you saw several varieties of cells crawling around as they went about their tasks. Some of these cells, such as the phagocytes, did not normally live at the site and had journeyed from elsewhere in the body to get there. This observation brings up an important point: before they can do anything, inflammatory and immune cells must first be delivered to the site by the bloodstream.

Their situation is analogous to an army that requires ships and railroads to transport their tanks to a distant battlefield before they can fight. This is an important principle of healing: an injured or sick region without adequate blood supply, especially if that place is of substantial size, can rarely heal completely. There must be a good supply line. This is the main reason a foreign object like the splinter inhibits healing: there is no blood vessel conduit that gets inside the splinter and thus no way to deliver cellular soldiers directly to the spot.

The bloodstream does more than transport phagocytes, immune cells, and cellular reinforcements to the battlefield; it also is the supply line for the third act of the drama, when healing means rebuilding. This requires energy, fuel for all the cells involved in the rebuilding process, as well as molecular building blocks to make new tissue. Those needed materials arrive at the site via the bloodstream, along with the oxygen that allows the cells to burn the fuel they need as they work. If there is no way to get the raw materials to the construction site, the cells cannot do their job. Plus, as is often the case, if antibiotics are needed to help the immune and inflammatory systems kill the bacteria, these medications also need the bloodstream to get to where they need to go.

A retained splinter is a simple example of what we term a foreign body. These things are notorious for slowing down or even preventing complete healing. Over time, the body often can get rid of a small foreign body like a splinter by remodeling the tissue around it in a way that forces it out. Sometimes this can happen with even larger foreign bodies. Like many of my colleagues, I have seen cases in which a deeply embedded object gradually worked its way out to the surface long after the injury that put it there. But we cannot count on that happening.

A retained foreign body contaminated with germs slows healing, but oftentimes the body can eventually heal around it even if it stays in place. If, for example, all the bacteria there either are killed or eventually die off, inflammation will fade and the third act in the healing drama can proceed, at least in a limited way. What generally happens is that the body quarantines the object behind a wall of tough, impervious scar tissue. This is not as good as getting rid of the object, but it is possible. The body's ability to accomplish this depends upon the size of the object and how contaminated it is with germs. A large, germ-laden object is very difficult to deal with in this manner.

Not all foreign bodies impede healing. This is a good thing, because these days we use implanted foreign materials all the time in medicine. In fact, surgeons learned over a century ago that they could leave stitches deep inside the body and the stitched-up area would still heal. These days we do much more than leave stitches behind. We can replace entire joints with new, artificial ones made of plastic and titanium. We can replace parts of the heart and blood vessels with grafts made of woven fabric and place so-called stents in small blood vessels to hold them open. We can even place electrodes into the delicate inner ear you saw in chapter 2 to help hearing.

These useful foreign bodies differ from those that cause problems in a key way—they are sterile, carrying with them no germs. When, as occasionally happens, such a surgically placed item becomes infected with bacteria, it is transformed into something very much like the splinter. It is extremely difficult to heal the area unless the contaminated foreign body is removed. Like the splinter of wood, an artificial hip has no nourishing meshwork of blood vessels to bring cells and supplies.

There are other ways besides hiding out in a retained foreign body that germs can find sanctuary from the body's defenses and delay or even prevent healing. A very common one is a collection of pus—dead germs, phagocytes, and leftover debris from their mutual struggle, as well as a few live germs. The body usually (although not always) can manage to wall this material off into an abscess and prevent it from spreading anywhere else. If all the bacteria inside the abscess are dead, and the abscess is relatively small, eventually the body will clean everything up. It does this by progressively making the abscess cavity smaller, breaking down the cells inside to their constituent parts, and absorbing the result.

If the abscess is a large one, however, and especially if there are still live germs inside, then the best the body can manage is a stalemate in which the germs are surrounded by vigilant sentinels of the immune and inflammatory systems that prevent them from breaking out and spreading. Such a situation never heals completely, and it is always a ticking time bomb for the body, because there is a risk the germs can break out and spread.

Sometimes healing can be delayed simply if there is a large amount of dead tissue that needs cleaning up, even if that material is not infected with germs. This can happen following what we term an infarction, a situation in which there has been a blockage to the blood supply sufficient to kill the cells that depend upon that particular vessel for their nutrients and oxygen. Eventually the cellular cleanup team takes care of all this, but if the infarcted area is large it can take weeks or even months for this to happen.

Not all dead tissue can be completely broken down, hauled away, and recycled into new tissue—bone, for example, can pose a problem. When a bit of bone loses its blood supply and dies it can persist, not doing its former job, and blocking complete healing. This can happen at a spot of previous bone infection or at a fracture site that has small fragments of bone that lost their blood supply.

In the previous chapter you read about how we can deal with most of these sorts of arrested or blocked healing by removing the pus or dead tissue. This act can be as simple as lancing a boil or as complicated as major surgery, but the principle is the same. Once the source of chronic inflammation is gone, the healing drama, arrested in the second act, can then move along to the third and final act. Unfortunately, not all causes of persistent inflammation are amenable to such a straightforward solution.

Chronic ear and sinus infections are common examples of places in the body in which smoldering inflammation can linger because drainage there can be difficult. You have already visited the middle ear several times and learned how important good function of the auditory tube is. If fluid builds up there, it is prone to become infected with opportunistic germs lurking in the region. The sinuses can present a similar situation.

Without sinuses our skulls would be very heavy indeed to carry around. Nature has lightened our load by providing our skulls with air-filled cavities—the sinuses. These cavities are very much like the middle ear. They are lined with the same kind of cilia cells that sweep mucus out their front doors and down into the nasal passage. Like the middle ear, if that drainage becomes blocked or just does not work well, chronic inflammation and infection is the result. The way we deal with chronic sinusitis varies and can involve a mixture of medicines to improve drainage and treat infection and surgical approaches to drain the sinuses, but the principle is simple—provide and maintain good drainage, and the local immunity you read about previously can keep the area neat and clean.

In all of these examples, persistent and chronic inflammation gets in the way of healing primarily because the normal healing systems are working at a disadvantage. If we make the contest fair by removing the pus or foreign body, the cells are free to accomplish their tasks and usually do so. These are easy examples. There are other examples of persistent inflammation that are more difficult to understand and explain. Whatever their cause, they share the property of interfering with normal healing.

Chapter 5 told you all about immunity, that marvelously tuned system that protects us from outside invaders, like germs, and possibly from rogue cells of our own that can turn into cancer. The most important thing the immune system must do is to learn to tell the difference between our unique selves and everything else, to distinguish between self and non-self. When confusion arises, the result can be the serious problem of autoimmunity, situations in which our immune systems attack our own tissues.

Autoimmunity very often leads to chronic inflammation. This will not surprise you, I am sure, after what you have seen on your various trips to inflamed parts of the body. Some immune cells attack directly anything they regard as foreign, and the antibodies other immune cells make flag for destruction whatever they think is an enemy. This process causes the release of the chemical messengers that are the fuel for inflammatory reactions—the swelling, pain, redness, and tenderness we can see with the naked eye—as well as the cellular events we need a microscope to see. The normal immune response has built-in regulators that switch it off when its work is done; with autoimmunity, however, that off switch is defective and confused, so the inflammation continues.

There are other chronic, generalized inflammatory states that are not truly autoimmunity, but, like autoimmunity, they are situations in which the body has great difficulty stopping what should be a self-limited process. You can think of asthma in this way. Although for most children the inflammation around the airways eventually improves on its own, indicating their bodies have some control over the cellular events, it may not entirely go away without the help of medications. There are also several disorders of the intestines, aptly termed inflammatory bowel disease, in which persistent, smoldering inflammation causes trouble.

All of these things, from retained foreign bodies to autoimmunity, slow down or even prevent complete healing, because the principal character in the second act of our three-act play—inflammation—refuses to leave the stage. I am sure it will be easy for you to guess how we deal with this situation—we get control of the inflammation. If there is a foreign body, like a splinter, we take it out. If there is an abscess that needs draining, we drain it. For many of the other situations, such as autoimmunity or severe asthma, we use medications that block inflammation.

We must be careful when we use these drugs, though, because the relationship between inflammation and healing is a delicate one. Inflammation protects and heals us, but when it is too severe or persistent, it prevents us from healing. When we try to tame inflammation with drugs, we strive for a middle ground, dampening the inflammatory fires enough to allow healing but not so much that the body cannot defend itself. It is a fine line to walk.

A common reason for many instances in which healing is delayed or blocked is reinjury. You can think of persistent inflammation in this way: the tissues in the inflamed site are never allowed to heal, because, on a microscopic level, the inflammatory cells just keep whacking away at their targets, even when it is no longer appropriate.

There are many other examples of how reinjury blocks healing. An itching rash that refuses to go away, for example, may really still be there because your child cannot help scratching it, causing new injury that itself itches. The continual runny nose of a child with allergies is really the same thing—continual exposure to whatever the allergen is, such as ragweed, reinjures the lining of the nose. Likewise, the child you read about in chapter 5 with gluten sensitivity could not heal his intestines until the intestinal lining cells stopped being constantly reinjured by the gluten in his diet.

Another useful example to consider is the one from chapter 8, your son's broken arm. Broken bones make for impressive injuries. The noise of the bone snapping can be easy to hear, and often the body part is bent out of its normal shape. The damage is also impressive on the inside, as you saw. There is usually a substantial amount of blood present in the tissues around the fracture site, especially if the bone is a large one or is one of the bones particularly rich in blood cell–making marrow.

As the cells around the fracture site get busy repairing things, they often need outside help. Sometimes fractures are what we call non-displaced—the edges of the break are still next to each other and all is in proper alignment. Fractures of the skull bone are commonly like this and will heal on their own without us doing anything. For many fractures, however, if we do not align the bones in the way we want them to end up, there will be a permanent deformity after healing is complete. The broken bone edges will nearly always knit together in some fashion, even if we do nothing, but they need guidance if the body part is to resume its previous good function. Humans have known this for millennia; bone setting is an ancient trade.

In a fascinating aspect of healing, the body is amazingly good at fine-tuning the ultimate bone alignment. In your son's broken arm, for example, it was not necessary for the orthopedic surgeon to get his arm perfectly straight before immobilizing it in a cast. The alignment, or the degree of angulation, can be off by a surprising amount, and the bone will eventually straighten itself out through remodeling.

What must happen is that the edges must be close enough together without wiggling around as the bone is trying to heal. If they are too far apart, the busy osteoblasts, the bone-forming cells, cannot bridge the gap. If the edges are unstable and move, newly formed bone is continually being reinjured. Each time that happens, a new wave of inflammatory messages arises, and the repair crew must start all over again.

I am sure you can easily think of many other examples where failure to heal is really caused by failure to allow the tissue a reasonable chance to heal. There is a good reason the first item in the list of things to do for an injured arm or leg is rest—leave it alone and let the healing cells do their work. Thus, a tennis player with a sore elbow who keeps playing or a typist with a painful wrist who keeps pecking away at the keyboard both repeatedly thwart their bodies' attempts to heal.

Both persistent inflammation and repeated injury explain many situations in which complete healing is inhibited. In both these situations the body's normal healing mechanisms, on the cellular level, are actively trying to get things right but find their efforts undone. They resemble somebody bailing the water from the bottom of a boat while somebody else is dumping water in; the boat will never be empty unless the second person quits working at cross-purposes with the first. There is another group of healing problems caused by an entirely different mechanism. In these situations, the healing process is not being continually sabotaged but is itself too feeble to get the job done. There are several reasons this can happen.

Sometimes the immune and inflammatory systems just do not work very well. Age can be one reason for this. Small infants have not yet gotten their systems completely up and running. By the time a child is a few months old, however, most everything is functioning at capacity. A practical result of this observation is that some vaccines do not work very well in small babies, which is why we wait to vaccinate them against many diseases. On the opposite end of the age spectrum, elderly people find their defenses running down after a lifetime of use.

Mounting a proper immune and inflammatory response takes energy. A child who is not well nourished can show decreased ability to do this, although in practical terms an otherwise normal child needs to be quite malnourished for this to become a problem. So parents should not worry that several days, or even weeks, of a poor appetite due to illness will affect their child's ability to fight off germs or heal a broken arm.

Very rarely, a child will have some intrinsic problem with her immune or inflammatory system or with one of the other aspects of tissue healing, such as bone repair. If present, this is usually something she is born with, although not always. The hallmark of such an inborn healing problem is that it is chronic—it is not something that comes and goes. So children like that will typically have experienced a string of illnesses or injuries from which they have difficulty in healing. We have specific tests for most of these conditions and nearly always can help the situation.

Additionally, as you have read, the body's defenses are multilayered, providing several avenues of protection that complement each other by working in different ways. Thus, a problem in one of these systems, such as local immunity in the lining of the respiratory tract, can be compensated for with the other components of the system working normally.

Tissue healing can also be blocked if a person is receiving one of the medications that dampen immunity or inflammation. This is more of an issue with adults than it is with children, since adults are much more commonly taking these sorts of medications, but it can be an issue for children because sometimes they are used in younger people. Some examples of these medications are chemotherapy drugs for cancer and what we call "immunosuppressive drugs."

The latter family of medications is actually intended to block immunity—it is our goal to create a partial immune defect. Examples of conditions for which we use them are people who have bodywide inflammation, such as an autoimmune disorder, or who have received organ transplants. As you read in chapter 5, the body always attacks an organ that comes from somebody else unless we partially handcuff the recipient's immune system to prevent it.

There is still another way healing can be disrupted or even prevented. Sometimes there are difficulties in getting the needed materials—cells, nutrients, and oxygen—to the spot that needs to be healed. All of these things must come to the inflamed or injured tissue by way of the bloodstream, so if there is some difficulty with that essential supply line, healing suffers. Children generally have excellent circulations. They are young, strong, and do not have bad habits, like smoking, or chronic health problems, like heart disease or diabetes, that can narrow or block off the meshwork of blood vessels needed to bring the building supplies to the cellular work site.

In spite of that advantage, sometimes a child's healing can be inhibited by problems with the circulation or by the fact that the tissue that needs healing is one that has a relatively poorer blood supply than other parts of the body. A not-uncommon example of this principle is following some sort of injury. Your son's broken arm was a common injury, one easy to fix. Unfortunately, children sometimes suffer more severe mishaps, injuries that can do more than break bones—they can injure blood vessels, too, or isolate body parts from their blood supplies. Surgeons who care for such children know that an important part of their job is to do what they can to ensure that the healing tissue gets a rich supply of blood. If it does not, the injury will not heal well.

In spite of all the wonderful measures nature has devised to help us heal, sometimes they are not enough—sometimes healing fails simply because it is overwhelmed. In a few of these situations the components of the healing process themselves, especially the blood clotting and the inflammatory systems, contribute to the difficulties.

Recall for a moment your very first microscopic adventure, the trip to your son's inflamed and infected finger. The tissues around you at that time were angry. The blood capillaries were engorged with blood cells. The cells that lined the vessels had pulled apart, creating gaps in the tiny pipelines that allowed, even encouraged, fluid and blood cells to leak out into the surrounding tissues. This leakage was a central aspect of the defense system because it allowed needed cellular reinforcements and blood components to reach the site.

On that trip, as well as the one to the broken arm, you also saw the blood-clotting system in action. You saw how nature has contrived a way to take a fluid—blood—and quickly convert it into a solid in places where patches and plugs were needed. The blood platelets, those bits of cellular dust, played a major role in that particular mini-drama; they provided an initial plug by joining hands with each other and then served as the base on which the scaffolding of the clot fibers could grow and weave its strands together.

At least as important as the platelets for blood clotting were the cells that lined the blood vessels. You first saw these cells when you noted the cobblestone pavement surrounding you as you traveled inside a blood vessel in chapter 1. Each cobblestone was a single cell. Compared to the action you saw in the finger—phagocytes crawling after attacking bacteria, second-echelon cells building support structures behind the phagocytes—the blood vessel lining cells appeared to be mere bit players. True, they did have the job of opening and closing gaps to let other cells through on the way to the battle, but that seemed merely like stage door workers helping the stars get in and out. But even though you could not see it, these lining cells, called endothelial cells, are central to how inflammation and blood clotting work. They do much more than open and close stage doors.

The infected finger had little bits of blood clots here and there, but chapter 8, the trip to your son's broken arm, was where you got an impressive view of how blood clotting works. As you saw, an absolutely essential aspect of blood clotting is that it happen where it needs to happen and nowhere else. The clotting system is aptly called a cascade, because it is a linked series of events, a chain reaction. These linked events have a series of control points, places where the chain reaction can be either accelerated or decelerated. The outcome is a tightly controlled clot, right where nature wants it.

In addition to limiting the clot to only where it needs to be, when the clot is no longer necessary, it must be broken down and taken away. A vessel highway that has been temporarily blocked by road construction needs to be reopened so that blood can flow again. This process, too, is highly regulated so that the clot is neither removed too soon nor left in place too long.

The endothelial cells, those seemingly boring pavement cells that line the blood vessels, are the masterminds of the blood-clotting system. They release substances that can start and stop the reactions that turn liquid blood to solid clot and back again. They modify and alter the molecules on their surface that are exposed to the bloodstream in ways that tell platelets what to do and where to stick and make plugs on their surface.

There is more—endothelial cells are also the masterminds of the inflammatory events you have seen in so many places. The coordinated cellular events are controlled by sequential release of all those substances that serve as chemical messages between cells. Some of these messages call cells to the scene, others fine-tune how the cells behave when they get there, and others are even responsible for the symptoms we feel, like fever and malaise, when we have an illness more extensive than a splinter in our finger. Many of these messages that regulate inflammation come from endothelial cells.

To the cells at the site, inflammation is like a powerful storm. The phagocytes and immune cells unleash potent weapons that, although effective against invaders, also damage or even destroy innocent bystander cells that are minding their own business. This is a sacrifice the body is prepared to make, since cellular losses and local damage can usually (but not always) be repaired later. Better to lose a few innocent cells than to allow invading germs to gain the upper hand and spread. You have seen what happens to the battlefield during and after the struggle, a scene reminiscent of the African proverb that reminds us that when elephants fight, it is the grass that suffers.

Like blood clotting, it is crucial to our health that inflammation is limited to where it needs to do its work. Sometimes the body has no choice in the matter—if the involved area is large, then so, too, must the inflammatory battlefield. Limiting the fight to a more confined area would not be a good idea. The more extensive the process, the sicker the child. There are times, however, when all of the components of the inflammatory process—the phagocytes, the cells of the immune system, and all of the substances released by these activated and angry cells—spread far beyond the original battlefield. The result is widespread activation of the inflammatory system in places where not only is it not needed, but where it can do significant harm. We have a name for this condition. We call it systemic inflammatory response syndrome, abbreviated SIRS, and it can be a very serious problem.

There are many things we do not understand about SIRS. When there is a huge attack on the body, a massive infection or injury, it is understandable that the resultant inflammation is equally massive. What is less clear is why a less extensive attack can do the same thing, and why this can happen in such an unpredictable way.

One of the mysteries of SIRS is why the same set of conditions in two different individuals can provoke it in one person but not the other. Genetic predisposition is probably one reason. This should not surprise us. After all, consider the condition of autoimmunity you read about. There is clearly a strong genetic component to the propensity in some people to have their immune systems become confused and attack their own tissues, which is what autoimmunity is.

This misguided immune response probably happens at least now and then in many of us, perhaps all of us. Generally we can snuff out the aberrant reaction and return to normal. Autoimmunity happens when the rogue cells break free of this control. The phenomenon of SIRS may well represent a similar situation; all those chemical messages, which should be exerting their effects at the proper place and at the proper time, somehow switch on the inflammatory system everywhere.

The bodywide inflammation of SIRS can have enormous consequences, most of which are the result of all those vessel-lining endothelial cells waking up and thinking they should do what they normally do at inflammatory sites—increase the vessel diameter, open up gaps to let out fluid and cells from the bloodstream, initiate blood clotting, and release even more substances that summon phagocytes. When these new phagocytes arrive, they let fly with their arsenal of weapons designed to destroy invaders. But in this case there are no invaders, so only the surrounding tissue cells get injured to no good purpose.

The problems a child who experiences SIRS tend to be worse in those parts of the body where there is a relatively large number of endothelial cells. From what we know about the syndrome, this is entirely predictable because endothelial cells are the principal actors. One place that is especially affected is the lungs.

If you recall your visit to the lungs in chapter 3, you remember that when you were deepest into the airspaces, in the alveolar air sacs, you were surrounded by a shimmering fountain of blood. The blood flowed all around you, separated by the thinnest of transparent membranes from the air sac where you lay watching. This structure let oxygen easily pass from the air to the blood and carbon dioxide travel in the other direction. All of those thin walls were covered, on the blood side, by endothelial cells. In fact, an enormous percentage of the total cellular mass of the lungs is made up of endothelial cells.

From what you have seen in the finger, the appendix, and the lung, you can now easily imagine what a widespread conversion of lung endothelial cells from a sort of docile wallpaper on the vessel walls into participants in inflammation could mean. The cells pull apart and open up gaps between them, allowing fluid and inflammatory cells to flood into the air sacs. Once there, the phagocytes and their friends unload the munitions they carry in their granular magazines. This injures surrounding cells, provoking even more inflammation. Worse, when the alveolar air sac becomes flooded with fluid, air can no longer get in, and the lung cannot do its job of exchanging oxygen for carbon dioxide. This is why nearly all people who contract SIRS have difficulty breathing.

The kidney is another organ that is particularly rich in endothelial cells, and SIRS causes major problems there, too. If you were to get inside your exploratory vessel and visit a kidney in the throes of such widespread inflammation, you would see the same thing—leaky blood vessels and marauding phagocytes. One vital job of the kidney is to remove body wastes from the bloodstream. Another is to maintain a precise balance in our blood between water and the various chemicals, such as sodium chloride (salt), which we need to live.

An inflamed kidney does not do these jobs well. Nature has provided us with quite a bit of reserve capacity in our kidney function—we get along just fine with only one instead of the normal two, for example—but SIRS affects every part of both kidneys. If severe, the result is serious or even dangerous imbalances in the chemicals in our blood.

One of the most serious things SIRS can do is launch the blood-clotting cascade everywhere. The endothelial cells mistakenly believe clots are needed, so they call down the platelets and set off the series of chain reactions you read about earlier. SIRS also sets off the chain of anticlotting reactions, so the entire bloodstream does not turn into a massive clot, but this, too, can be a problem because the anticlotting mechanisms will dissolve clots everywhere, even where they really are needed, causing bleeding. Both the unwanted clots and the bits of dissolved clots circulate throughout the body, often causing even more problems when they lodge in important small vessels, closing them off. It is a very difficult situation to treat.

Healing from cancer can present an additional set of problems. As you have read, cancer is not really one disease but rather a family of diseases that share the property of out-of-control cellular growth. It may be that our immune systems can root out some cancers when they are composed of only a single cell, or perhaps a few cells, but we are not entirely sure about how that works, or even if it does. But once cancer is established, the body is relatively powerless against it.

It is true there are rare but well documented cases of cancer apparently regressing or even disappearing on its own. We do not know how that could happen, but the extreme rarity of this fortunate result emphasizes how poor our defenses against it generally are. Realistically, we cannot heal from cancer without help from surgery or chemotherapy. If those measures work, then we heal the ravages of the therapy itself using the systems you have read about already.

Ideally, healing restores the tissue that was sick or injured to its previously normal function. Certainly this happens with virtually all the illnesses or injuries your child experiences. Sometimes, though, this cannot happen. For example, the places where your child's phagocytes and immune cells fought it out with an infection or an injury may remain as scarred as any battlefield. The third act of the healing drama, in which cellular debris gets carted away and the repair team reconstitutes the area, may still leave residual damage that is beyond repair.

Organs that have been inflamed and then have healed may not look normal under the microscope, even though they look fine to the naked eye, and those regions may not be able to do their normal cellular work. Nature, in her wisdom, has provided children with extraordinary healing abilities. She also gave them enormous reserve, backup capacity, in most of the major organs. Thus a child can usually get along just fine in spite of carrying a scarred but healed spot of lung, liver, kidney, or many other organs.

This chapter has been about some of the ways healing can fail. Ultimately, of course, all healing fails because we are all mortal beings. Yet this extraordinary system works well in nearly all of us, especially children. Nature has been tinkering with tissue healing for a very, very long time, even for her time scale. The evolution of healing goes far back in our cellular memories. The final chapter tells you what we know about how and when the amazing things you have witnessed first arose.

· 12 ·

Healing and the Tree of Life

$\mathcal{H}$ealing is as old as life itself. In fact, without it, life would be almost impossible. The world is a dangerous place for all creatures, posing continual threats to survival. Some ability to ward off these attacks and mend the injuries they cause is a necessary skill for all living things, from the simplest organisms to the most complex. Without that ability, the struggle to survive long enough to reproduce and carry on the species would be far more difficult than it already is. This is undoubtedly why all of the processes you have seen and read about in this book extend eons back into our evolutionary past.

Even single-celled organisms like the amoeba, one of the simplest of creatures and one that has been on Earth for more than a billion years, have ways of fighting off the advances of hostile germs around them. Amoebas, like other primitive, single-celled organisms, have the ability to release substances that are toxic to the germs but not to the amoeba.

Once creatures with more than a single cell appeared, organisms could have some degree of specialization; that is, cells in the organism could divide the labor of existence among them. This process allows cells to devise increasingly better ways of doing their jobs. Thus, for example, in our bodies we have cells in the intestine that are proficient at absorbing nutrients. Nearly all the cells in our bodies are highly specialized in this way.

Scientists have been able to discover, far back in our evolutionary past, examples of organisms that have already assigned specific cells to the task of fighting off invaders, particularly bacteria—germs. A very

189

special variety of amoeba, called the social amoeba, provides a fascinating example of how this can work. This creature lives as a single-celled organism most of the time, fending for itself, like other amoebas to which it is related. But when environmental conditions deteriorate, a multitude of them band together and form a sort of slug. In an astonishing display of "out of many, one," a large group of these organisms meld together into a single creature. The kinds of things that can cause this phenomenon are a decrease in food supply or other environmental changes.

When this slug forms, the amoeba cells, previously entirely independent, begin to divide up the tasks necessary for them to go on living. They form a sort of commune of common interests. As part of this process, certain cells are deputized by the others to patrol the entire commune and protect the inhabitants from attacking germs and toxins—in effect, they become primitive phagocytes. Once they begin to devote their time to patrolling for invading germs, they even acquire better ways of killing the invaders when they find them.

Interestingly, phagocytes very much resemble amoebas in their ability to crawl around independently, unattached to any of the tissue scaffolding around them. Like the cells the social amoeba appoints to protect the new community of cells, phagocytes have a specialized job. Our phagocytes have much more sophisticated weapons for doing their job than these amoeba sentinel cells, but the principle is the same. We should not be surprised that our phagocyte-amoebas have learned a few tricks over the past billion years.

Chapter 5 discussed how the immune system does its important work. We distinguished in that chapter between two arms of the immune system: the humoral system, meaning things dissolved in the blood, like the antibodies, and the cell-mediated system, meaning those cells that can kill invaders on their own. There is another way to divide the components of the immune system, one that tells us a great deal about our evolutionary past. These other two large categories are called innate and acquired immunity. In your travels throughout the body you have seen examples of each.

Innate immunity describes those aspects of immunity that all humans are born with. These are in the genetic toolkit we inherit from our ancestors, and we do not need vaccines or anything else to awaken our ability to use them. When you visited the lining of your son's auditory tube, his middle ear, and his upper airway, you saw part of the innate immune system in action.

Phagocytes, those hunter-killer cells you have seen in so many of our scenarios, are very ancient components of innate immunity. The nineteenth-century Russian scientist Elie Metchnikoff first discovered phagocytes and even identified and studied them in very primitive creatures— ocean starfish. So we have inside us, protecting us from harm, a defensive army made up of cells very similar to those that swam in primordial seas a billion years ago. The social amoebas of today still exist, of course; you might think of them as those members of the amoeba family that were perfectly content to remain amoebas over the intervening years.

Our modern phagocytes carry deep, ancestral memories of their enemies, especially germs. Hard-wired into their genes is yet another molecular signaling system that does not use antibody flags to identify a suspicious particle as a germ: ancient struggles have imprinted themselves in the phagocytes so that the surface properties of many bacteria trigger a phagocyte attack. This is not as powerful a system as those we have developed since, but this aspect of innate immunity allows us an additional measure of protection from the microbes our forbears have fought many times in the past.

There is another aspect of innate immunity that helps phagocytes do their job. It is the complement system you read about in chapter 5. Like antibodies, complement proteins are substances dissolved in the blood, but unlike antibodies, complement proteins do not need to learn what their target is—evolutionary memory has told them what to do, which is to attach themselves to invaders and help phagocytes destroy them. As you recall from chapter 5, the complement system is made up of a family of proteins that is activated during inflammation in a chain reaction, cascade manner, which is similar to how blood clotting works. Once activated, pieces of complement proteins signal to the phagocytes what to attack by attaching to them. Complement is also one of the most potent chemical messages for calling new phagocytes to the scene.

As with phagocytes in starfish, the complement system is another example that shows how far back into our evolutionary past innate immunity extends. Starfish have complement. Primitive worms do, too, as well as many other creatures alive today who also swam in ancient seas. The complement system uses existing templates, taken from our collective genetic memory banks, to identify attacking bacteria. This works because many bacteria share attributes that have not changed over time. But it is not an optimal defense system, because some things have changed and have done so in ways that can bewilder our phagocytes. Still, complement can be a quite effective defense system; after all, billions of organisms lacking our own more sophisticated immune weapons rely upon complement as a key aspect of their cellular defenses, and they continue to flourish on Earth.

Thus, innate immunity has been around for a very long time. Another observation tells us how very ancient innate immunity is: it is not unique to the animal kingdom—plants have it, too. Like animals, plants have germ enemies—bacteria and viruses—as well as parasite enemies. Plants do not have the kinds of free-ranging defender cells, like phagocytes, that can roam around the plant looking for invaders, but plants are not defenseless. When plant cells are attacked by a germ, they release messages that tell the surrounding cells to make substances to limit or halt further invasion by the germ. The ability to do this is of great interest to agricultural researchers, because they are always on the lookout for ways to make crops resistant to disease.

Innate immunity is very useful, but adding acquired, learned immunity to its powers is even better for healing and survival. How did we acquire that ability? Astronomers speak of the Big Bang as a shorthand way of describing the origins of the universe. There are examples of sudden, similar, game-shifting changes in biology, after which nothing is ever the same. In what has been called the "big bang" of immunology, somewhere around 450 million years ago acquired, or adaptive, immunity appeared. Sharks and their relatives are the most primitive creatures still alive today that first benefited from this immunological leap.

The key to the big bang of adaptive immunity was the ability of the immune system to learn who the enemy was, to be able to adapt on the fly to new information about what was self and what was non-self. To do this, the immune system needed to be able to generate the huge number of antibody varieties needed. Besides the unique antibodies, adaptive immunity also conferred upon organisms that possessed it new kinds of special cells—lymphocytes—that could specifically identify invaders. Adaptive immunity truly changed the game, giving organisms that had it a major advantage. The world is an extremely complex place, with many possible varieties of attacking foes.

Adaptive immunity is a way for our body to develop new defensive tricks. It has a disadvantage, though, when compared with innate immunity: we cannot pass on to our offspring what our own immune system has learned. Our children must begin the learning process for themselves. It is true that, at birth, a mother gives her newborn baby a several-month supply of antibodies to launch her child into life. These antibodies represent the sum of what the mother's immune system has learned during her lifetime. This maternal immunological helping hand wears off soon, though, after which the child is on his own, helped only by the innate immunity all humans possess.

Recall from chapter 5 that we get all the different antibodies we need by a process called clonal selection. Deep in our lymph nodes, our immune systems are continually churning out millions and millions of potential antibody-producing cells, as well as the T-cells that direct them. Each one is coated with a randomly generated version of an antibody. These cells sit there, waiting.

What the lymphocytes are waiting for are tissue macrophages, those scavengers, like tiny magpies, that diligently bring to the lymph node the assortment of things they have collected during their travels throughout the body. In chapter 5, you followed one of these wanderers when it made its way to a regional lymph node after scooping up a bit of the vaccine your friend's son just received. The macrophage was bringing it to the node to see if anybody was interested in buying it.

As they arrive in the lymph nodes, the macrophages display their wares to the lymphocytes. They do this by sticking the things they have found in a special place on their surface, like a shopkeeper's display window; they behave very much like a salesman showing shoes to a customer. Only in this case, it is a single shoe offered to a host of customers; it is like looking for the Cinderella who fits the shoe.

When there is a fit, that is, when a particular antibody is a good match for what the macrophage is selling, then that lymphocyte is selected. It reproduces itself into more cells just like it, as well as making more of that antibody. The cells that do not show a match die off, to be replaced by new ones that line up to see what is on offer by the next traveling macrophage that comes along.

The great leap forward, the key part of the big bang for immunity, was the ability to generate all the millions upon millions of varieties of antibody molecules. This ability, at first glance, violates one of the standard rules of cell biology, the so-called one gene, one protein rule. The rule states that it takes a single gene, a unique piece of our cellular inheritance, to make a single protein. The gene is the template—the mold—to make the protein. We get a gene from each parent to make all the proteins we need. An antibody is a protein. If each of us has only two antibody genes from our two parents, how can we make the millions of specific varieties of antibodies?

Around the time sharks evolved, there came an evolutionary breakthrough that solved the puzzle. Nearly 500 million years ago, in some primordial sea, an archaic ancestor of today's sharks was infected by a virus. This was a quite ordinary event, one that had been going on for eons— viruses are ancient, too. As luck would have it, this particular virus gained access to the shark's reproductive germ cells and changed the DNA. This meant that whatever the virus did to the shark's genetic material could be passed down through the generations to future sharks. More than that, whatever future creatures ultimately evolved from this clone of archaic sharks also had the altered DNA.

Some viruses insert themselves into the DNA of the cell they are attacking. This particular virus had that ability, as do some viruses today. That virus had another ability that some viruses still have—the capacity to mix up the DNA of the cell they are infecting.

This special gene-swapping capacity happened to land in a region of the shark's germ cell DNA that controlled the synthesis of the proteins of what would become antibodies. This was a fantastically useful ability for all the creatures that were to follow that shark, because it allowed an animal to take the two antibody genes from each parent and scramble them around into many millions of combinations. Once this sort of gene shuffling could be done, all the needed diversity of antibodies was possible. Ever since then creatures with this ability, like us, have been able to learn from attacks by germs. We, and every other animal descended from that primordial shark, can make specific antibodies to protect us the next time that particular germ comes around.

We know many of these things because the actual genes—the sequences of the genetic code that pass from generation to generation—are highly conserved over time. That means the genetic sequence for our complement proteins is very similar, virtually the same, as that of lower organisms. The same goes for antibody sequences. Once nature devised a system that worked, she stuck with it.

These insights into the evolution of inflammation and immunity tell us a great deal about where healing came from, and how, from amoebas to sharks to humans, nature has learned new ways of protecting us and promoting healing. Over the eons, however, nature has also apparently lost a few skills in healing. She has made us so complex that it is very difficult, when we are injured, to put us back together again exactly the way we were before. Complexity is good; it has allowed amazing things to evolve. But all higher organisms have paid a price for this complexity, too.

As an example, consider planaria, a form of flatworm about a quarter-inch long. It is a favorite both of scientists who study growth and healing and of high school biology teachers looking for ways to intrigue and inspire their students. One reason for the planaria's popularity is that it is easy to grow and study, but another reason is that planaria can do incredible feats of healing. If you cut a single one of these creatures in half, each half grows an entirely new half to replace the lost portion, and the resulting two planaria are completely normal. Even a fragment as small as an eighth of the original worm can regenerate an entirely new worm.

The healing skills of planaria are an excellent introduction to the notion of stem cells, a subject of intense interest to scientists who study all manner of healing. Animals begin life as a single cell, rapidly dividing into two, then four, then eight, and so on. Under the microscope, these first few generations of cells look identical. Very soon, however, they begin to distinguish themselves from one another in a process called cellular differentiation. Cells destined to become cells of the nervous system, for example, develop the specialized functions of the nerves, spinal cord, and brain. Likewise, the primordial intestinal, heart, and all other organ-specific cells soon can be distinguished from each other.

The differentiating cells soon begin to look different from each other under the microscope. They also display on their surface specific sets of proteins that mark them as future nervous, digestive, or other system cells. The way this happens is that cells, as they differentiate into whatever their ultimate task will be, undergo an intricate set of what we call gene activations—certain genes are turned on, but a great many are permanently switched off. This means that, although it is true that every cell in our body carries identical genes and has the same DNA, most of the genes are inactivated. The cells use only the genes they need to do their particular job.

What we call a stem cell is a primitive, undifferentiated cell that retains the capacity to develop into any kind of cell in the body. Planaria, it turns out, are composed of nearly a third stem cells. When needed, an injured planarium can call upon this stock of stem cells to differentiate into whatever is needed to make a new organism. Planaria and creatures like them pay for this ability to regenerate by remaining primitive in their capabilities.

Reaching the complexity of higher mammals requires intense specialization of the body's cells. Like specialists of all sorts, though, our own specialized cells know more and more about less and less. Can we improve healing by getting some of our cells to forget their specialized function, to de-differentiate into more primitive cells that might learn new tricks, new functions? We have evidence that this can happen when we look at cancer cells. As part of their rogue, out-of-control nature, cancer cells often switch on genes that the normal process of differentiation had turned off. So we know this is possible. Might we get cells to do this in a controlled way? Better yet, can we find new stem cells anywhere?

It took some time for medical researchers to realize that, even though our bodies are fully formed, there are still some stem cells hiding here and there inside us. These are probably not the truly beginning stem cells, those that can differentiate into anything, but they can still learn to perform a wide variety of functions. A good portion of healing research these days is devoted to devising ways to enlist these lurking stem cells into coming out of hiding and forming new tissues.

We already make routine use of the stem cells that can differentiate into blood cells. Years ago researchers found that such cells circulate normally in the blood. They are very rare in comparison to all the other cells in the blood—certainly you did not see any of them during your expeditions through the bloodstream—but medical scientists have learned how to identify them by spotting the protein markers they carry on their surface.

Once we could identify them, technology solved the problem of how to harvest them. We have machinery that can, when blood is run through it, sort the blood cells into different groups based upon the markers on their surface. We can even transplant these collected stem cells from one person into another. A stem cell donor simply lies on a bed with a small tube in a vein in his arm that directs his blood through the machine; afterward the blood goes right back into the donor.

Each pass of a stem cell donor's blood through the machine yields a few stem cells. Simply passing the blood through again and again over several hours yields enough stem cells to put into the veins of someone whose bone marrow has failed. Once inside the recipient's body, the blood stem cells repopulate the bone marrow and become normal, functioning bone marrow cells. The person who donated the stem cells quickly makes more to replenish those he donated.

Blood stem cells have moved slightly down the differentiation pathway, meaning they can only become blood cells and not, for example, nerve cells. But blood stem cell donation is a model researchers hope some day soon to apply to many other kinds of healing. As of this writing, the debate over using embryonic stem cells—the truly universal cells that can become anything—continues. There are significant ethical issues about where these cells might come from, a debate beyond the scope of this book. But many believe these cells could restore all sorts of damaged tissues, especially in the brain and spinal cord. We are not sure yet how we might do this or what sorts of stem cells we might do it with, but it is an area of intense research that I think will sooner rather than later provide practical therapy options to help tissues heal that are injured beyond the body's capacity to repair them unassisted.

In this book you have journeyed far and wide throughout the body to see how healing works. You have seen that the inner universe of children's bodies, though microscopic, is a vast and intricate place. It is made up of an entire society of cellular citizens, each of which has a special job to do. The result of all these cells working together is to realize the total entity that you recognize as your unique child. Illness or injury is a disruption of this cellular society, and healing consists of restoring it again to working order. As I wrote at the beginning, it is an astonishing and miraculous thing to watch. By now I am sure you agree.

Suggestions for Further Reading

$\mathcal{I}$n this book, we have considered topics ranging widely over the broad medical fields of microbiology, immunology, physiology, and pathology. Interested readers can find more detailed information about these subjects in standard texts available in all medical libraries and many general libraries. Such books do assume a certain amount of background knowledge in the reader, typically at least that of college courses in the sciences. The most helpful books for general readers are those written for medical or nursing students rather than those for fully trained physicians. I have listed the latest editions of several of these books, but older editions (from the last decade or so) could be useful, too; texts like these are quite expensive, and libraries may not have the latest edition.

There are also many useful online sources of information on these topics. However, readers should be cautious in their use of these; unlike well-accepted textbooks, online sources may be written by authors of unproven expertise or by those who have nonstandard viewpoints. The best way to avoid these potential problems is to stick with online sources from widely recognized authorities or organizations. And the medical texts will be easier to understand if you first consult some of the online sources listed below.

ONLINE RESOURCES

http://www.nlm.nih.gov

This is the site of the National Library of Medicine, a division of the federal National Institutes of Health. It is a public resource, available to all. It is a huge site, but its home page is well organized into sections directed at general readers and health professionals. It has a good search function. It maintains an excellent list of nontechnical articles written for general readers about current medical news, as well as many other topics. It is an excellent place to search for articles in medical journals about particular questions you may have, although the articles themselves are often highly technical.

http://www.aap.org

This is the site of the American Academy of Pediatrics. The academy is the professional organization of America's pediatricians and is thus the official voice of doctors who specialize in the care of children. The site has many useful and reliable articles on general issues regarding children's health and healing, which are available to anyone. The scientific articles, however, are accessible only to members of the academy.

http://www.mayoclinic.com

This is the public information site maintained by the Mayo Clinic. The home page contains a frequently updated list of articles about current medical topics. There is an alphabetical list of original articles written by Mayo personnel about a wide range of health topics. The search function is excellent. The information is mostly geared toward practical answers to questions about particular diseases, but many of the articles contain good explanations of what is happening inside the body during healing. There are also general descriptions of how the body works, such as this one about the brain: http://www.mayoclinic.com/health/brain/BN00033. Many of the articles provide reference lists for further reading, and the cross-linking between different articles on the site is well done.

http://nobelprize.org/educational_games/medicine/immunity

This is the official site of the Nobel Prize committee. It contains a good general description of how the immune system works. The site also has a wealth of excellently written pieces about many aspects of the medical sciences, particular those related to Nobel Prize winners. If you are interested in learning more about the immune system, this is a good place to start.

http://www.gluegrant.org/inflammation101.htm

As you have learned, inflammation is key to both disease and healing. This excellent site is written by scientists at the famed Massachusetts General Hospital. The whole purpose of the site is to make research into inflammation understandable to the public, and it does a good job of this. It provides what they term "Inflammation 101," a brief, illustrated primer in how inflammation works. There are also many other helpful features on the site; for example, the "frequently asked questions" section is particularly good.

http://www.nlm.nih.gov/medlineplus/mplusdictionary.html

A good medical dictionary is an essential aid for understanding what you are reading. This site, provided by the National Library of Medicine, is a good one. Besides just defining the words, it also has a tutorial explaining how medical words got their meanings. This allows you to understand many additional medical terms without looking them up.

BOOKS

Brooks, George, Karen Carroll, Janet Butel, and Stephen Morse. *Jawetz, Melnick, and Adelberg's Medical Microbiology*, 24th ed. New York: McGraw-Hill, 2007.

This is a venerable text used by generations of medical students to learn all about bacteria, viruses, and other things that cause infections, as well as how our bodies fight them off. Much of it is understandable to anyone who has studied something about these topics in college courses.

Delves, Peter, Seamus Martin, Dennis Burton, and Ivan Roitt. *Roitt's Essential Immunology*, 11th ed. Hoboken, NJ: Wiley-Blackwell, 2006.

For years Doctor Roitt's book has been the most widely used immunology text for colleges and medical schools. The best parts about the book's many editions have always been the outstanding illustrations, which are colorful, vivid, and easy to understand. The text itself can be a bit dense. A good way to use this book is to read about the basics of immunology elsewhere (such as the Nobel Committee's Web site listed above) and then to look at Roitt's illustrations.

Guyton, Arthur, and John Hall. *Textbook of Medical Physiology*, 11th ed. Philadelphia: Elsevier Saunders, 2005.

Guyton's physiology textbook is also an old friend to several generations of medical students. In fact, it is one of the most influential medical texts ever written. Although it is aimed at medical students, anyone with a college course or two in biology will find much of it understandable. Medical physiology is the science of how particular organ systems work, so the book is organized into chapters about the heart, kidneys, digestive system, and so on. There are also some good opening chapters explaining how body cells work in general.

Kumar, Vinay, Abul Abbas, and Nelson Fausto. *Robbins and Cotran Pathological Basis of Disease*, 7th ed. Philadelphia: Elsevier Saunders, 2005.

To a physician, pathology is the study of abnormality—tissues and organs behaving in ways they should not. Dr. Robbins published the first edition of this pathology text thirty years ago, and, like the other books in this list, it has become a standard. The opening chapters about how cells work and what happens when they do not is very readable for most general readers. The section on inflammation is excellent, although it is a bit complicated for general readers. The section on cancer is also good, and it is easier to follow than the section on inflammation. The bulk of the book, like most pathology textbooks, is organized by specific diseases and body parts. The latest edition includes many stunning color photographs and illustrations—earlier editions aren't as colorful.

Index

abscess, 12; poor healing of, 176; treatment for, 13, 157–58
acetaminophen, 112
acquired immunity, 81; origins of, 193–94
adaptive immunity. *See* acquired immunity
adenoids, 22
airflow in lungs 42
albuterol, 52
allergy, 94–95, 122; treatment of, 97–98
alveolar sacs, 45–46
amoeba, 189–90
anesthetic, 159
antibiotic, 13, 30, 70
antibody, 29, 144; origins of, 194; production by B–cell, 76, 193; structure of, 78–79
antihistamine, 97, 123
aorta, 7, 128
appendicitis, 68–69
appendix, 63, 66; origins of, 70
artery, 5
asthma: allergies in, 95; inflammation in, 52, 178; key derangements

during, 48; prevalence among children, 38; psychological aspects of, 169; treatment for, 38, 51–53, 170; triggers for, 38, 98
auditory tube, 22, 25; in otitis media, 26; special attributes of in children, 27
autoimmunity, 82, 84, 87, 104, 178
autoantibodies, 83, 104

bacteria, 23, 132; in appendicitis, 66–68; in the normal intestine, 61–63; in otitis media, 27
basal metabolic rate, 162
Benadryl, 97
beta–cells, 85
bile, 60, 64
biopsy, 104
blood cells: counts of, 150, 153; red, 8, 93–94, 131; white, 8
blood clots, 11, 132, 137, 158, 182
blood supply, importance of for healing, 175, 182–83
bone: calcium in, 130, 138; callous formation, 139; cells of, 129; cortical, 129; marrow, 130–31, 154;

About the Author

Christopher M. Johnson, MD, is a physician trained in pediatrics, infectious diseases, hematology research, and critical care medicine. He is a former professor of pediatrics at Mayo Medical School and director of pediatric critical care medicine at the Mayo Clinic. He is the author of more than one hundred medical research papers, as well as two other books for general readers: *Your Critically Ill Child: Life and Death Choices Parents Must Face* and *How to Talk to Your Child's Doctor: A Handbook for Parents*.